The pleasure shape

Techniques, Tips, Spells and Analysis of human seductive behavior and sexual health.

Seducing is an art and like all art, seduction is learned and developed. Although for many it is an innate gift, today we are telling you details that may be interesting to both men and women. Some people think that the art of seduction is just one more complement because everything will depend on the physique, not on whether they are beautiful people or ugly, but that physical attraction between the two occurs; other people consider that everything depends on the lip with which one introduces himself to the person that interests him and how he can play with it; the most romantic consider that it does not matter the physique or the lip because when you find that person you do not need more words.

Table of contents

Introduction. 3

Tips to attract a man 4

How to seduce a man?...6

Signs that indicate whether a man is good in bed...13

Games in bed to share with your partner...20

Do you want to buy your first dildo and you do not know which one to choose?.................24

Mistake you should not make when you are conquering a man. 26

How to provoke a man sexually. 28

Keys to female body language. 32

How to seduce a woman...33

Mistakes you should not make in bed. 41

Dirty things to say to a girl to get her wet with 42

Woman who are good in bed do these things...46

Most effective techniques for female orgasm..49

Tricks for women to agree to oral sex. 52

How to talk to my partner to have a threesome? 56

Painless anal sex..59

Most extravagant fetishes..61

10 tips for masturbation as a couple 63

How to masturbate a woman correctly 65

How to masturbate a man...68

Love moorings- Easy and Powerful. 72

How to increase libido..86

Tricks to increase your sexual desire today...89

Foods to Produce More Sperm 90

Sex in the car: the 6 best positions to do it in the car. 93

The 10 sexual positions to get a deeper penetration. 96

Tips for watching porn as a couple..100

Introduction.

I thank and congratulate everyone who has acquired this set of information, it will be of great use if what you want is to improve conquest tactics, The form of seduction is a book that will solve the problem of those readers who seek to improve skills of seduction, this book will show you what behaviors to avoid when conquering the person you find attractive and therefore want to conquer, as a personal experience I have always been interested in the art of seduction, in my case women are such beings wonderful and beautiful, we humans are very interesting beings and we have a high level of reasoning, which is why seduction techniques are infallible if applied correctly, this information will help you lead a life without fear of failure, however failure It is always and will always be the first step to success, it will benefit your way of thinking as well as understanding the attitude and behaviors of people Regarding the subject of seduction, I suggest you read the book and take a few minutes to let yourself be involved in the world of seduction, do not wait any longer.

Human beings have the ability to communicate and express our feelings, either with female or male body language. When words are too many or missing, we can resort to these non-verbal strategies, such as female or male body language.

The idea is that, from now on, you are aware of what your face, your body and your gestures communicate.

Seducing is an art and like all art, seduction is learned and developed. Although for many it is an innate gift, today we are telling you details that may be interesting to both men and women.Some people think that the art of seduction is just one more complement because everything will depend on the physique, not on whether they are beautiful people or ugly, but that physical attraction between the two occurs; other people consider that everything depends on the lip with which one introduces himself to the person that interests him and how he can play with it; the most romantic consider that it does not matter the physique or the lip because when you find that person you do not need more words.

Be that as it may, we interact differently with the people who attract us and although sometimes we are not aware, seduction strategies are put into play to get their attention and / or to keep it.

Tips to attract a man

- FACE

Unquestionably, the face helps us to convey our non-verbal emotions, since it is the first reference to a conversation.

Therefore, it is necessary to know what we are expressing while we speak or when we are in silence.

For this reason, it is necessary to talk about some factors and places of the face that are present at a certain moment when interacting with others, especially when being with a man.

- LOOK

"The eyes are the mirror of the soul", pay close attention to everything they express!

If you have a date, it is better that you opt for a day in which you are not too tired so that your eyes do not express fatigue or sadness.

Also note, before your departure, that your eyes are clean. If you like to wear makeup, highlight it naturally.

If you think that makeup is not for you, do not worry, your seductive look will shock him. Focus on making eye contact with the man you like; If he's attracted to you too, this will make him nervous. You will know it easily because, when a man stares into your eyes it is because he is also interested in you.

Remember that the idea is to seduce him and not intimidate him too much, be subtle!

- EYE MOVEMENT

If you find it very difficult to look at him carefully and fixedly in the eyes, you can intersperse your gaze or do it a little sideways.

Turn your head a little to the side, as if you are observing something else, do not stop there and look at it with slightly narrowed eyes while you smile.

A mischief would be great.

- EYEBROWS

Eyebrows frame our eyes and are very important in facial harmony, as they are impossible to ignore. It is convenient that you pay attention to them; If you have them very thin, opt to let them thicken a bit, and if they are too thick, it would be ideal that you manage.
Remember that everything in excess is bad. When you are speaking or listening to him, try to be aware of the movement of your eyebrows. You can be interested, in front of something that he is telling you, raising both eyebrows a little and adding a smile or gesture of astonishment. But you should not be serious, since he will think that you are not interested.

- MOISTURE YOUR LIPS

If you have chosen to apply lipstick, use a soft tone but that enhances your lips, this will attract the attention of the man you like. Now if you didn't apply any lipstick, no problem. For both cases, when he is talking to you, and while you are looking at him intently and intently, choose to moisten your lips a little or bite them gently.

- THE POWER OF SMILE

The power of a smile is decisive for the success or failure of your date, since it says a lot about your personality. The smile is usually related to positive emotions or well-being, but this is not always the case. Below you will find the main types of smiles and what each one expresses.

How does the smile affect when it comes to flirting or falling in love?

the smile affects in terms of love and can facilitate the situation when flirting with someone.

1. You will be more attractive.

2. You will enhance your sexual attractiveness.

3. You will sound sweeter when speaking.

4. You will transmit more confidence.

5. You will have more to choose from

The smile is the best way to know if a person is shy or not. The individual who has a shy or reticent smile is characterized by slightly tilting the head, not showing too many teeth and slightly averting the gaze. Although at first it may not seem like the best way to captivate you, the truth is that this type of smile is extremely attractive, since it conveys a certain aura of mystery. Within this category, the so-called "conquering smile" could be included: it is one in which the gaze is diverted, to recover it again furtively.

How to seduce a man?

Most men are attracted to women who take care of themselves in every sense of the word. We speak of respect for oneself, trust and security, that they dedicate time to their image. We are not talking about thinness but about taking care of the image that is transmitted, enhancing those parts of yourself that you like from the physical aspects such as your qualities and abilities.

Femininity is a weapon of seduction by itself as well as confidence and security, they are aspects that cannot be missing. A woman who is sure of herself before others and especially before that person who attracts you, is much more attractive than that doubt. On the other hand, we also find the other side of the coin, there are men who are attracted to shyness and insecurity in a woman, they like to be the ones who dominate the situation.

"Easy is boring" A phrase that seems unforgettable and is that for many men it is necessary for women to pose a challenge to attract their attention, so playing difficult can be one more point to add to your attractiveness but beware, there is a point where the difficult becomes tiring and not all men are governed by the same.

Women like the smell of masculinity of men, for many it is not necessary to use cologne or perfume because their own smell can become the best sexapil but many men enjoy the perfume of women. Find the perfume or scent that defines you, the one with which to drive a man crazy so that whenever he smells it he becomes a permanent memory of yourself.

Confidence in yourself can be your best weapon. Recognize the beauty in you, enhance it and feel powerful, sexy, nothing better than knowing how much you are worth so that others also want to discover it.

Do not deceive yourself: it is possible, on certain occasions, that your obsession with that person can cause you not to see things as they really are. If you come to a situation where you are not calm and you do not know what the other person is feeling, it is best to move on from that person and move on.

Happiness: this point is closely related to the previous one, with this what we mean is that your happiness is above anything and that you should not change it for anything.

Seduction goes beyond a passionate kiss, a frantic caress or a suggestive phrase; learn more about how to seduce a man in bed below.

It is an act of persuasion, an art that, despite being innate, in most people, has various tactics and tricks that are developed over the years and, above all, with experience.

Now, when it comes to knowing how to seduce a man in bed and how to drive a man crazy in bed, not all women are clear about it and, sometimes, they need more than the simple advice of a friend.

Do not lose sight of any of the tips that I bring you below and begin to fully experience intimacy as a couple!

CONQUER HIM FIRST!

Before proposing to seduce him, turn to conquest as the key to enjoying a balanced intimate encounter. In which a strong desire is fused with feelings that go beyond mere passion.

But how to do it? It is very simple!

Read the following list and put your plan to work.

- ACTIVATE EACH OF YOUR SENSES

  Inciting him to desire you is the first step in knowing how to win over a man who is still undecided and fascinate him, even before they have an intimate encounter.

If you want to know about assertiveness in sexuality, read this article by redalyc

The key to doing so is to activate or stimulate your senses with small details that, due to their subtlety, are very effective. Take a look at these tricks to make him fall in love and dare to put them into practice!

  1. Sight: Men are basically visual; therefore, it is important that you always make a good impression. A good look that mixes sensuality with delicacy, she will love it! Because you will leave a lot to her imagination; in the same way, it is ideal that you take care of your makeup and hairstyle, since they also pay attention to these two aspects. If you add a seductive look or smile to the above, he will fall at your feet!

2. Smell: On the one hand there is personal hygiene, to which you must pay special attention and, on the other hand, the smell with which you want to identify you. Try to use a mild but strong scent, so your guy associates you with him and cannot get you off his mind.

3. Hearing: In this case your best allies will be words; A good conversation that achieves an adequate connection between the two is crucial as a prelude to any subsequent more compromising situation. The talk can be accompanied by carefully selected music for the special occasion; Your man will not be able to resist your charms and the best thing is that he will conceive you as a woman who can offer him much more than a night of passion.

4. Taste: You could fascinate him with a delicious dinner, followed by an excellent wine and, why not, some sweet kisses. You will have the opportunity to surprise him and get his taste buds addicted to you.

5. Touch: The friction or small touches, almost pretending that they were without intention, will make you lose your head! Think about it, play it strategically and you will see its positive reaction; but always remember to make it look casual.

SECURITY AND TRUST

These two words are essential to know how to seduce a man in bed, and they are the winning duo to make him value you and know how to make him see you as the most special woman in the world. Show him your firmness, your convictions, and your certainty regarding all aspects of life, from the sentimental, professional, to the sexual plane.

Speak without fear, defend your points of view, and make him see that you have great power, that you feel comfortable with your body and with your way of being and thinking. But most importantly: make it clear that you do not depend on anyone to be happy and feel fulfilled!

MAKE ME SEE YOU AS A CHALLENGE

Do not let me take you for granted; men love challenges and, therefore, if they conceive you as a challenge, they will love you; learn more about the Mirror Method.

Do not make things easy for him, give him the opportunity to fight for you and to have you fully. Never forget that if you put yourself on a silver platter, he will quickly lose interest in you.

Then, the best thing is that you choose to play a bit difficult and wait for the right moment to give him what he deserves.

SEDUCE HIM IN BED

Now that you know the tactics to conquer him without failing in the attempt, it is time for you to know how to seduce a man in bed and thus guarantee a high degree of excitement and infinite pleasure. Without further ado, here are the tips, one by one, to help you persuade him intimately.

Use your imagination!

Surprise him! Make her feel incredibly special thanks to your seduction tricks.

Although the traditional never fails, it is time for you to try new methods to enchant your boy in bed. There are thousands of options, it is a matter of analyzing your partner's tastes a bit and that is it!

A sexy costume or lingerie, an erotic dance, an oil massage, a game of truth or dare with questions to get to know your boyfriend better; are some ideas to inspire you and revolutionize it.

TAKE THE INITIATIVE AND BET ON SPONTANEITY

Men love women to take the initiative, do not wait for your partner to always be the one to start flirting or courtship.

It is time that you put aside prejudices and show yourself as a determined lady, who has all the control and who has all the skills to handle the situation.

If, apart from taking the initiative, you add a bit of spontaneity to the matter and give fluidity to the meeting, without inhibitions and with an open mind to the possibilities, he will not want to let you go!

Provocative attitudes are quite momentous; rediscover the sensuality that lives in you and enjoy, together with your man, an unforgettable experience.

1. THE RIGHT ENVIRONMENT

To seduce him you must try to ensure that the environment that surrounds them is correct; that is, a quiet space where they can laugh, talk, express themselves and have fun without worry.

The light, the aromas and the romanticism will make him feel comfortable and ready to be enchanted by you.

2. ROLE PLAYING GAMES

Any boy is crazy about his wife being playful, daring, and wild. The previous moments are essential, and for this reason I advise you not to discard role-playing games and understand that men, like you, have many fantasies, and fulfilling a few or all of them, there is nothing wrong.

On the contrary, it will strengthen the confidence and seduce him accurately, it will no longer be a problem.

LET YOURSELF BE OBSERVED
Let him turn on the light, if he wants to, but do not stop him from looking at you and stroking you. Seduce him with gentle movements or shudder! This will be a plus to steer him in the right direction. Help him to travel your body, guide him with your hands and gaze at him; This will cause him to crave you madly.

3. KISS HIM

A good kiss seduces, falls in love, and activates all desire sensors! Your man will feel that you want him, which is an excellent seduction strategy and even more so in bed.
Do not just think about kissing her lips; the neck, chest, abdomen, among other erogenous zones, are ideal to provoke it, disturb your mind and activate all your nerve endings!

4. MAKE HIM WAIT

How to seduce a man in bed? Make him wait! Not only will he increase his passion, but he will fight to get you. His arousal will increase significantly, and he will focus only on you. While you wait, you can delight him with an overdose of kisses, caresses, massages, well thought out phrases to fall in love to raise his temperature or a sensual dance. The rest, I leave it to your imagination!

5. TAKE A HOT WATER SHOWER WITH HIM

While taking your shower, invite him to participate and, in a matter of seconds, without much effort, you will have him at your mercy and absolutely seduced and in love.
Think about it! He will love being with you in such a situation. Just make sure you unleash her desire to the fullest!

6. TALK ABOUT SEX, DON'T BE AFRAID!

It is assumed that before becoming intimate with someone, it is appropriate to have prior knowledge; This, to be clear about the tastes of the other and thus please him more in every way.
One of the most relevant but most taboo topics for talking as a couple is sex.
Do not be afraid to talk about your sexual preferences, it is something very natural and information that you can use later to your advantage.

7. UNDRESS HIM SLOWLY

When you think the time is right, start removing some of her clothes, slowly.
Start with his shirt, twist it, touch it, offer him another glass of wine, make him want
you! and then continue to get rid of her clothes. With this attitude, he will know your
intentions, he will give in to your game and he will be happy to participate in it.

8. Try trying new positions; that routine does not extinguish the flame of passion.
Remember that there is the Kama Sutra and there are thousands of techniques that you
can use to please your man. Innovate, renew your sex life, and earn points with your
partner!

9. Don't complicate yourself in bed; Remember that perfection does not exist, so do
everything possible so that both you and your boy enjoy the moment, the pleasures
and forget about limits.

10. In the morning, in the afternoon, at night or at dawn, it is always a good time to get
into the art of seduction! Break the established rules and provide your man with
unique experiences that he cannot forget and that haunt his thoughts, when you are
not around.

11. After a massage or gentle caresses, take it hard; This change in pressure will alter him
in a positive way and he will be encouraged to correspond to you also passionately, so
you will know how to seduce a man in bed.

12. Expand your sexual repertoire and make each encounter both special and different; try
fellatio, even if he does not tell you, and you will make him incredibly happy. With
this practice you will realize that learning how to seduce a man in bed has never been
easier!

13. Move while you brush it! The way you move, I leave it to your consideration; The important thing is that you do not stop and keep a good rhythm; You will not regret it and your boy will thank you!

14. Sell it, handcuff it or tie it up; use these tactics and arouse more than just your curiosity. Mystery and doubt will captivate you; Let him get into your game of seduction, walk away, and get closer, kiss him, caress him, and provoke all his bad thoughts.

15. Temperature changes are a particularly useful and effective tool for your boy to lose control. An idea that can work wonderfully, due to the intensity, is to pass an ice cube over his back or chest and then warm the area with your breath and mouth; Give it a try and you will see the results!

16. Do not forget that your partner also needs tenderness, sweetness, and attention. Shows of affection are essential to strengthen the relationship both on a sentimental and sexual level.

Signs that indicate whether a man is good in bed.

There is a lot of talk about what details are characteristic of men who are good lovers and are good in bed. For example:

What signals do they send? or how do they behave? If you are meeting a boy and you have just asked yourself this question, be attentive because in the following lines you can find the answers to these questions and thus you will get rid of doubts.

1. Dance well

Many women love dancing, and this can be a great aphrodisiac to get in tune and finish body to body in the room with that man. This not only includes a good "striptease", but some dances awaken our most intimate and passionate instincts.

This is what Dr. Peter Lovatt, a psychologist at the University of Hertfordshire (UK) thinks. He decided to carry out an investigation in which he recorded 15 male forms of dancing so that later a group of 55 women of different ages will visualize them. The results showed that the John Travolta moves in "Saturday Night Fever" are the most stimulating for females.

Also, many women claim that dancers are good in bed. This is what a study by the British company Phones 4U concluded, as more than 80% of the women surveyed assured that there was an association between a good dancer and good movements in bed. What is more, up to 50% of women said they check a man's movements before going to bed with him. That is why many women think that Latin dances are exciting.

2. He is adventurous.
Adventurous men also seem to be good lovers and good in bed. Because they are people who enjoy new challenges and look for exciting moments and adventures in their life. This can also be a great aphrodisiac, as these types of people want to try new and unconventional experiences. Something that in the long run can keep the flame of passion alive in the relationship. Intimate relationships without taboos are much more pleasant.

3. Kiss well
If you have already made out with him and have noticed that he kisses like angels, he will probably make you have a good time in bed. If he kisses well and knows that he kisses well, it is because he surely has a lot of experience and is a person who gets carried away by the situation. It is spontaneous and is not guided by conventions.

Logically, this is not 100% infallible, but if that person kisses you with passion, it means that he likes you and it turns on your physique (and possibly your mind). The chemistry you can have with that person who kisses well is a good beginning to move on to the next phase with certain guarantees of success.

4. Has high self-confidence.
In intimate relationships, self-confidence is the key. A man who is confident in his sexual performance and knows that he is good in bed will give you incredible moments. On the other hand, a shy person in this environment will surely not be able to let go and enjoy sexuality so fully. In addition, self-confidence is one of the qualities that make us more attractive.

5. Makes you feel like an attractive person.

When you find someone, who makes you feel like a spectacular and incredible person, the degree of intimacy between the two increases. Some women feel insecure, and to fully enjoy themselves, they need the other person to make them feel special. Words are not enough to achieve this.

6. Has a proactive and ambitious attitude.

Ambitious and proactive people are always on the go and generally enjoy better overall health. Think about it. Would someone who spends the whole day playing video games be better in bed or someone who worries about not spending a lot of time sitting, goes out with friends and does sports on a regular basis? People who have an active life generally enjoy better health. That is why they perform better in virtually any physical activity.

7. he is creative.

Creativity can be a good indicator that this person will make you feel extraordinary things. If he has an active life and is healthy, cares about you, uses different ways to make you feel someone who gives off attraction, has confidence in himself and is creative, probably this man has something that you might like. The reason is that by not having to dedicate time and effort to follow a "script" everything happens in a much more fluid and spontaneous way.

DIRTY WORDS AND PHRASES THAT YOU CAN USE IN BED

1. It feels so good I want to scream.

Although it is not a very risqué phrase, if you say it at the exact moment and with a sensual voice, you will surely turn him on a lot.

2. I love how your tongue feels there.

In addition to being a sensual phrase, it is a way of indicating what you like so that they get to know each other better.

3. You are a bad boy.

Many men (and women) like to role-play and like to be made to feel like dirty, bad boys, so if your partner likes it, whisper it while you pet him.

4. Squeeze me harder.

Another way to tell your partner what you like. Tell him to squeeze some part of the body that you like the most and use a suggestive and sensual voice so that it is also exciting.

5. I have been waiting and imagining you all day.

A phrase that you can use right in the foreplay. Besides being overly exciting you make him feel good and desired, that always increases the excitement.

6. It is so big it hurts but I want more.

In the moment of greatest climax, you can say something like that. It is a dirty phrase that is extremely exciting. Do not forget to tell him with a sensual tone.

7. Put it in now.

After a lot of foreplay and the intensity has increased, you can say this dirty phrase to him that is sure to raise the temperature even more.

8. I feel very wet.

This phrase is exciting because you will make him feel that he is doing a good job. That will make you work harder and increase your safety.

9. It is getting hard.

You can say this phrase with a very sensual and suggestive voice while you caress it. It will surely increase the temperature even more.

10. You make me very horny.

You can whisper this into her ear when they are just for playing or she is just kissing you. These are magic words to go to the next level.

11. I am touching myself right now.

Use a few dirty phrases to message throughout the day. You will surely get them excited and when they see each other, there is already a lot of intensity.

12. I am not wearing underwear today.
This is another phrase that you can send to your partner before meeting. If you feel more daring, you can accompany it with a suggestive photo. Of course, remember that you must have a lot of confidence in him and that he will not misuse your photos.

13. I want to scream; it is so exciting.
During climax you can whisper this in her ear. Especially if they are in a forbidden place or where you cannot yell a lot, it is a phrase that helps raise the temperature.

14. I have fantasized about this moment all day.
Some words are ideal to ignite the spark. This phrase can be useful for that. As soon as you see him and they start with foreplay or kissing, tell him in a sensual voice.

15. Call me a bitch.
Some dirty words to turn on the temperature, surely many find it the most exciting.

16. Scratch me hard.
Some dirty words also work for you to indicate what things you like. A little harsh treatment many like. If hers is even more intense, let him know.

17. I want to lick your whole body.
Imagine saying this dirty phrase to him in the middle of a formal dinner. Something discreet to the ear that makes them excited and ignite the spark of passion.

18. I want you to target it now.
If you want to go from the foreplay to full action, you can say this phrase so that he understands it clearly, it is also overly exciting.

19. If you look at me like that, I get too hot.

Another way to excite your partner either before or during foreplay to make him understand that you want to go further.

20. You are thinking about what to wear today and I am thinking about how to take it off.
You can send her this message in the morning if you do not live together and make her smile for the rest of the day. If you see each other at night, surely, he will not resist your charms.

21. Take off my clothes.
A strong and firm phrase to go to the next level. Depending on the tone of voice and sensuality you use, it will be even more exciting.

22. You will get me there soon.
When you are in a very intense moment of your intimate relationship, you can say several dirty words to excite him even more.

23. I cannot take it anymore; we must do it now.
This is the kind of phrase you can use to go from foreplay to full action. Surely it will cause a lot of excitement.

24. You are so sexy.
A short but very sensual phrase that excites anyone. Whether you send her a text or voice message or use it when being intimate.

25. I want this for myself every night.
Although it is a somewhat more romantic phrase, it can also work to raise the temperature if you say it at the exact moment with the most sensual voice you have.

26. You do so well.
You can say something like that when you feel comfortable and to let him know that what he is doing you like; in this way he gets to know you more and excites him.

27. Go harder.
Another dirty phrase to say in bed. You will surely be able to excite him. Say this phrase in your ear and you will see that the intensity will increase.

28. Touch me here.

Said this phrase with all the sensuality and at the precise moment, it is more than dirty, very subtle but it can be as exciting.

29. I want to eat you whole.

When you want things to get more fiery, throw this phrase with all your determination and you will see that it works.

30. Bite me there.

Remember that to a large extent, that these dirty phrases work, they depend on your tone of voice and your sensual attitude.

31. I love the way you move.

If in addition to saying something dirty you want to make him feel good, say this phrase. If he feels confident, they tend to become more accommodating and caring.

32. Stay inside.

With as much sensuality as you can, say this dirty phrase to turn him on. It will surely excite you a lot.

33. I am coming, it's so delicious.

Either in the ear or yelling, you can repeat this phrase at the moment of greatest climax. Rest assured that it will excite him a lot.

34. Make me what you want.

By message or in person, this phrase always elicits reactions.

35. You are bad, you have behaved very badly.

If you want to be a little rougher, use this phrase to turn him on and take the relationship to a more intense side.

36. I am a very bad girl.

Playing and role-playing or playing the role of bad guys tends to turn them on a lot. Try this phrase and show off all your sensuality.

37. I like to feel your tongue all over my body.
A statement and phrase that is sure to turn you on. Plus, it's a great way to let it be known that you are doing something you love.

38. You do it so well and you make me feel so rich.
A dirty phrase to continue the excitement. The important thing is the attitude and the tone of voice to make it make a big impact.

39. I love when you get hard.
This dirty phrase tends to be liked by most men who like to hear things like that. So, seize the moment and say it in a sensual way.

40. What you do makes me feel extremely hot.
If they like to hear dirty phrases during intimacy, take advantage of letting them know what you like and at the same time excite him even more.

Games in bed to share with your partner.

Games in bed to share with your partner.

1. Sexual temperature
One of the classics of games in bed is playing with the sensations of our body. To do this, it is simply necessary to grab an ice cube or have a hot drink.

It is possible to apply ice directly on the body of the person we want to stimulate or put it in the mouth for a moment (as with a hot drink) so that when practicing oral sex or licking the partner the sensations are different thanks to the cold tongue or hot.

2. The detainee

Another of the classic erotic games consists of handcuffing one of the members of the couple so that he cannot move. In this game, a stoppage or capture is usually simulated.

One of the two members of the couple is tied hands (and feet in many cases) and is at the mercy of the other person who is responsible for giving pleasure. This situation is very stimulating for many.

3. Dice game

The game of dice is a variation of the previous one. It consists of the two members of the couple being assigned different numbers.

One the two even and the other odd. Then a dice is thrown and the person who wins is the one who will be tied for 5 minutes and will receive the pleasure of the couple.

4. Sex flavors

If the sensations of cold heat can be very pleasant, so can the flavors. There is nothing better than being with the person you love and delighting the palate with chocolate, strawberries, or ice cream.

The taste of each person can change, although some classics are smearing parts of the body with chocolate and cleaning them with the tongue. Also eat strawberries and champagne with the partner in an erotic way. The important thing is not to use your hands but everything else.

5. Oil massage

Massages are always pleasant and relaxing and are ideal for increasing sexual arousal and creating an ideal climate for sexual intercourse. The massage can be carried out in the same bed, where the person who receives it must be comfortable face down.

There are different types of oils with different aromas that produce different sensations. The touch, smell, and feel of the oil can be very invigorating, and a massage is ideal for foreplay in bed.

6. Sex bomb

The sex bomb is a juice in bed that causes a dynamite of pleasure. It is a simple game, which consists of taking a clock and setting a time interval in which it is not allowed to enter. If, for example, the time without penetration is 20 minutes, only caresses, kisses, bites, etc., are allowed until that stipulated time has passed.

7. Choose a piece of paper.

A game that can be very erotic and can excite your senses. It consists of taking two jars or jars (for each of the two) in which to put a series of pieces of paper. On each piece of paper, different verbs are written that have to do with sexual and exciting acts, for example, suck, lick, bite, etc. In the other bottle will be the papers with the written parts of the body. The combination of the two pieces of paper will tell you what you should do to your partner so that they feel great pleasure.

8. Blindness

Another mythical game is that of blindfolding, because when one cannot see, the other bodily senses are intensified. The operation is simple; blindfold and let the couple do their job to satisfy us. Imagination plays a fundamental role in this game, which is ideal when combined with the detainee's game.

9. The battle

The bed can be turned into a fighting ring with this game, where you don't have to be violent, but it can be fun. The two members of the couple must undress and hold a cushion with which they must start a battle. It is not about hurting but about having a good time. This can lead to a relaxed atmosphere that can end in love rather than war.

10. What does my mouth taste like?

This game in bed is ideal to combine with the game of blindness. Well, when one of the two members of the couple is blindfolded, then the other places different foods in his mouth: chocolate, ice cream, strawberries, liqueurs, cream, etc.

The goal is for the person who is blindfolded to guess what the other person has in their mouth. If it is not correct, then the person who was not blindfolded will smear his body with the food and the person who has lost has to lick it and clean the body without using his hands.

11.STRIP POKER

If your partner likes card games, strip poker is one of the ideal sex games for you. It is about playing poker as you normally would, but in this case the loser of each round will not have less chips or money, but something more sensual: he will be left without a garment.

To make this sex game sexier, the winner can decide which garment his partner will remove. Both of you dress for the occasion and add accessories that count as a garment, such as socks or ties. If they do not know how to play poker, they can play 21 or another simple card game they know.

12 BEER PONG EROTIC

If your partner likes card games, strip poker is one of the ideal sex games for you. It is about playing poker as you normally would, but in this case the loser of each round will not have less chips or money, but something more sensual: he will be left without a garment.

To make this sex game sexier, the winner can decide which garment his partner will remove. Both of you dress for the occasion and add accessories that count as a garment, such as socks or ties. If they do not know how to play poker, they can play 21 or another simple card game they know.
Golden Rule! Always try something new.

Although it is not exactly a sexual game, the best recommendation to get out of the routine and continue having sex full of love, pleasure and fun is to try something new (as simple as it may be) every time you have an erotic encounter with your partner.

How to do it? It is not difficult. You just must add something different in each sexual encounter so that none are the same as the previous one: from wearing new lingerie that your partner does not expect and you are already wearing, buying a lubricant that surprises her at that moment or an oil to give her an erotic massage. If you have never done so, it is the perfect time to buy a sex toy and the clitoris sucker may be the best to enjoy as a couple.

Other ways to surprise your partner and add something new without spending a single penny are to propose one of the sexual games on this list, do it in a different place than the bed, try a new sexual position or even add a very sexy touch with something who have not practiced before such as anal sex, petting, or exploring techniques to reach orgasm together, such as the coital alignment technique.

Do you want to buy your first dildo and you do not know which one to choose?

Before buying any sex toy you must first think about things like: how do you want it? What type of stimulation do you prefer? What size is best for you? And if you are going to use it alone or as a couple? Think about some guidelines of how you want your new vibrator to be, since it may be that with so much offer you will complicate yourself.

Choosing a vibrator is not easy, I tell you from experience, considering that there are more and more options that we can find, different sizes, different shapes, and even different functions, I am going to help you make a good choice.

Next, I will present a list of possible with important aspects that determine the purchase of some type of vibrator.

Are you looking for a vibrator to stimulate the clitoris?

Not everything that vibrates is going to be perfect to stimulate the clitoris, there are some whose shape allows it to better reach all the female folds of this little point of pleasure. I recommend you buy those that are waterproof, rechargeable, easy to use, and with different intensities of vibration.

Do you want a vibrator to stimulate the G-spot?

The vibrators that curve upwards are perfect for exquisite G-spot stimulation. These vibrators with the slightly curved upper end easily find the G-spot and produce incomparable sensations, but if you don't want to, you stimulate your g-spot without type penetration, the ideal is that you buy vibrating bullets, hopefully rechargeable, in addition, they are cheaper than a vibrator.

Do you want a discreet and silent vibrator?

Then choose those that have rechargeable batteries and not batteries, they are usually quieter. Also avoid those made of plastic; silicone vibrators allow discreet use in all circumstances.

Do you want to always carry it with you?

So that you never lack fun anywhere you go, choose the vibrators that fit perfectly in your hand, some have wireless control, allow you to change the intensity of the vibrations, they are ideal for masturbation, to use as a couple during penetration and to stimulate the clitoris.

Do you want to stimulate clitoris and G-spot at the same time?

Vibrators with this double function are a revolution of sensations for women. I recommend that you buy them with a rechargeable battery, because they only last one use and they sound quite loud, these are the most expensive vibrators, but they are the most complete.

Do you want to use a vibrator during penetration?

Then choose the vibrating rings, they are incredibly fun since they have a double function, for men and for women; The man places the ring on the penis and takes it to the end, the ring is turned on and with it a small vibrating bullet, and each time penetration occurs, the bullet will stimulate the woman's clitoris. If, on the other hand, the bullet is placed facing downwards instead of upwards, the stimulation will occur in the testicles in men, and in the anus or perineum in women. If you want to play with it before penetration, you can place it on your fingers and give stimulating massages on the penis or the external part of the vagina (Clitoris). Most of these vibrators are not disposable, they can be used multiple times; once they are done using it, washed it, and can be used again until the battery runs out. I do not know the first rechargeable vibrating ring, they all come with batteries. An important fact! If your partner ejaculates very quickly, buy a vibrating ring that puts pressure on the penis, they are elastic.

Mistake you should not make when you are conquering a man.

It can be complicated for many women who have no idea how to attract the man they like, and for years we have resorted to the advice of friends, without being completely sure that it works.

Some of the feminine behaviors when attracting a boy are negative and even absurd, which causes an effect contrary to what is sought. Here we leave you some of the mistakes that you may be making and that is why you have not yet found the right man.

1. Exaggerate your behavior.
When you are trying to conquer the heart of a boy, the best thing is that you are you, do not pretend to pretend something that you are not. If a joke does not sound funny to you, do not turn up the volume on your laugh as he will think you're acting and you're not authentic. Do not try to be too nice or always available.
2. Play dumb.
The best thing is that from the beginning you show your true personality; A serious mistake that some women make is to act sweet and somewhat silly, thinking that a man will like that, but if what you are looking for is a serious relationship, it is best to show your intelligence and the best of yourself.

3. Talk excessively.
We know, when you are with the boy you like, nerves appear and for fear of an uncomfortable silence you cannot stop talking, and this can become annoying. A good tip would be to let him speak; listen to everything he has to say.

4. Play hard,
In a relationship you need the interaction of both: if you like him, there is no point in making you inaccessible; If he asks you out and you are always busy, there may come a point where he gives up trying. It is true that men like to conquer women who are not available all the

time, but if you get to exaggerate the only thing you will achieve is to get them away from you. Everything with limits.

5. Look for commitments.

If you are starting a relationship, the most advisable thing is that you go slowly, that you try to get to know your partner before looking for something very formal and demanding a commitment too soon, the only thing that you will achieve with that attitude is to push him away. Either way, you better take the time to get to know him and see if he's also the person you've been waiting for.

6. Be very cloying.

When we like someone, we do not want to lose sight of them and we need to know how they are all the time, but you must understand that everyone needs their space and, if you do not let them breathe, sooner or later they will end up moving away from you. It is fine if you show your interest, but always with measure, if you are not going to overwhelm him.

7. Make up excessively.

Cosmetics were invented to help highlight your beauty, but when you cover your face with one layer of makeup over another, what you reflect is a great insecurity and this can be counterproductive in the long run. If you ask that man be natural and original, then you must be willing to deliver the same.

8. Pretend you like something.

If you don't like soccer or video games, don't pretend to show that you have extensive knowledge about it. For some strange reason, many women when they find out about the tastes and preferences of the guys they want to conquer, they try to convince them that they know a lot about the subject, but if it really is not your thing sooner or later, he will find out. The best thing is that, if you are interested, you start to question it; You will give him the opportunity to talk about what he likes and he will feel more comfortable with you.

9. Show off your attributes more.

Trying to attract the attention of a man by wearing provocative clothing may work in the beginning, but you are sending him the wrong signals. Nothing better than a self-confident woman, who shows her seductive side with clothes that flatter her, combining it with a charming attitude and a good sense of humor.

10. Lying about your age.

Many women are not ready for the moment when they are asked their age, except for those who are confident and content with themselves. You must understand that if someone likes you, it is because of you, not because of how old you are; those prejudices are already in the past. Be honest, it is for the best.

11. Contain your appetite.

When you go out with a man to dinner at a restaurant, it is best that you order what you want and you know that you are going to eat, do not try to look like a little bird that eats little; Either way, at some point he will realize reality. You fool no one by eating just a salad and a glass of water.

12. Provoke their jealousy.

It is true that when a man sees you talking to another, his instinct awakens and tries to gain your attention, but if you do it frequently only to make him angry and arouse jealousy, you will end up killing his interest and everything will end in a resounding failure.

How to provoke a man sexually.

You may just want to have fun with a guy you like, or have fun with your boyfriend or partner, if you want to give an exciting touch to your life or relationship with your boy, here I show you step by step what to do.

1. A good perfume

It is a highly effective and simple way to make a boy horny. Ideally, you should use some essence that you know you like. But if you're not entirely sure, use the essence of musk, which is a perfume that signals the brain to associate the aroma with sex.

Above all you should avoid aromas that are very heavy or strong (the musk is strong, but it is the only exception), and even worse those granny aromas. Apply the perfume behind your ears, on your wrists, and a little on your neck.

3. How to warm up and excite your boyfriend with a set of lips.

Another thing a man cannot resist is seeing a woman bite her lips. Just by biting them and using a lipstick and shine for the occasion, you will make sure he cannot stop thinking about your lips.

If you combine this with some killing looks, you will have it eating out of the palm of your hand. you will be ready to devour it, but you are not that kind of woman who says it directly, so far, you've only sent her very strong signals.

4. How to turn on your boy in your underwear.

The most important thing is that you do not wear your grandmother's panties, you must wear some that are shiny, thready. There is one thing men love, and very few can resist: seeing your underwear slightly above your jeans when you bend down or sit down.

5. How to light a man by talking to his ear.

One way to incite without even touching it is to whisper at the hear. You can take advantage in some conversation to tell him something tempting, or flirtatious. Always use a soft tone of voice, you should feel your breath nearby while using a warm and sensual tone. Only up to this point, if you do it right, he will be begging you to go to bed. Examples include:

You look so handsome (sexy, cute, provocative).

What do you want us to do now?

Do you want me to do something to you?

If you do not have it in front of you, you can try it over the phone, or by chat, you can insinuate yourself by sending it some provocative photo, or you can make some live video letting him see your neckline a little. Men are fascinated by photo and video seduction games. You can also try some insinuating text message.

6. Let him know that you are hot.
If it knows you are hot, you are finally going to warm it up. So, if he touches you in a way that you like, or said something you like, let him know. And you can let him know by whispering in his ear as we already saw. Do not beat around the bush, when you find yourself in this situation say something like:

You do not know how much I want you right now.
In my mind is only what I want you to do to me today.
Based on his reaction, you can heat up the environment more by saying a few dirty words to him.

7. It is time to play.
If at this point you have not managed to get him to bed, it is time to reinforce the signals a little more, in a more obvious way. And here I want to detail one of the things that you will not be able to resist. It is about touching his knee subtly while watching a movie, either in the cinema or on the couch, and then going up and down his thigh with your hand. In less than you expect, it will be begging you to touch other parts.
Of course, if you decide to go to the movies, it's not a matter of going any further, but it's an excellent opportunity to leave it wanting in seconds.

8. Dancing and touching it.
This point is simply to get to the same as the previous point, but by a different way. If you do not like movies, or watching movies, you can try dancing, it's an excellent opportunity to put their bodies together, and start fiddling. It is also not necessary to go to a nightclub, they can do it at home or in theirs (in fact it is recommended).

You must move naturally and take advantage of the songs in which they can bring their bodies closer. Let him take control, putting yourself on the submissive side will excite him a lot. You know men love asses, so take advantage of this to subtly (very slowly) put their hands on your ass. I assure you; he will love it.

When things get better, bite it in the ear. Making out (that is what I call the kissing and caressing game), it's very important to accentuate your ear or neck. His mind will fly, and he will want you to bite and lick other places. Followed by a simple kiss, it will be the prelude to an exciting night.

9. Going up and down the thermometer
So far, you must have achieved your goal by now if or if. But let's give it a few extra taps so he never forgets you.

Making temperature changes is very exciting, so when you remove the T-shirt, ingest your chest by drawing a long line, and then blow subtly over that line. This change from hot to cold will make him crazy.

10. Take off your clothes.
When it is time to undress, you must keep getting their attention, and for this you don't have to acquire the skills of the girls from the nightclub on the corner.

Just play some sensual music and use gentle body movements while taking off your clothes, this way you will keep your level of excitement extremely high.

11. How to warm a man using his fantasies.
Consensual perversion never hurt anyone. With this you will be able to give it an additional flavor that you will both enjoy as long as they agree. If he is interested in exploring his perverted side and you want to accompany him, they will enjoy it like never before. Never judge it, they are just fair, you do not have to feel uncomfortable either. Good communication is important.

Do not focus too much on the missionary's position, you will both get bored. Try different things while changing positions. When you are on top of him, face your breasts with your hands, this fascinates most of them. Try the 69 especially, both win.

And to close with a gold brooch, shower together, maybe it is the start of a second round, you know... And if they did not, they will have closed a spectacular night.

Keys to female body language.

Going out to conquer and flirting with guys is quite easy for some and quite difficult for others. But, contrary to what many people think, it has nothing to do with physical beauty, but rather with that innate flirtation that we carry within and the security and confidence that we have in ourselves. We have that person we like right in front of us and we get nervous, we get blocked and we do not know how to act. So sometimes we need to know some tricks to seduce a man that can help us at that time.

In any case, remember that the art of seduction also includes the other and the chemistry between you, however we leave you a selection of 9 tricks to seduce a man that will help you play your cards and make him fall in love instantly.

Here are the keys to female body language to keep in mind…

Play with hair.

I am not telling you to constantly touch your hair, do it when he is talking to you: run your fingers through your neck and then between your hair, play with him as if curling it, remember to be looking at your boy!

Whisper into her ear

 As you watch the conversation progress, you can gently approach her and say something into her ear; when you do, you will be entering their intimate space. Tell him something funny or something from the environment that you do not want anyone else to hear; when doing so, rub his ear a little, this will drive him crazy.

Touching the neck

 You can caress your neck a little and stretch it a little up or to the sides, gently, or simply rest your hand on the neck while you look at your man; you will inevitably notice him.

How to seduce a woman

Many women are attracted to large men, this is what some have called the "Hulk technique", the fact that you can offer comfortable arms and chest in which to shelter can become a great advantage because the feeling that is offered is security and protection.

Many men believe that one of the best techniques for seducing a woman is by approaching her and becoming her best friend. Probably, on some occasions this works, but there are also many men who consider that this type of technique is not only a risk but that it is doomed to failure, if they see you as a friend, they do not see you as anything else.

What do you think about the depressed technique? Approaching a woman and telling her your sorrows may be an aphrodisiac for some, since they will want to take care of you and pamper you, but for other women it can be completely the opposite and turn off their desire, they can listen to you but nothing more.

Although being smart and a "nerd" in adolescence may not be attractive, in adult life intelligence and culture are qualities that attract attention. Many women want their men to have a "bad boy" edge but also that they can offer them something else, that they can impress them. Although many think that chivalry has gone out of style, it is something that surprises all women, alike. the vast majority in a positive way and if it is negative, you are also getting to be unforgettable because few people remember having that kind of detail nowadays.

Humor and laughter is one of the most sought after qualities, consciously or unconsciously, in a partner. The newspapers are full of sad news, nobody wants to add more sadness to their life but everyone wants to be able to laugh, have fun and forget everything together with someone. Knowing how to make a person laugh and laugh at their jokes is an extraordinary incentive.

TIPS TO ATTRACT A WOMAN

1. Learn to identify your qualities.

Before the girl you like, you must show yourself how you really are, but you must learn to highlight your best attributes to get her attention. You must eradicate security and confidence, but without appearing arrogant.

If any weakness of yours comes out, try to disguise it through a joke, so that both of you can laugh at yourself, they love this! However, don't spend too much time talking about your weaknesses, change the subject.

When I tell you to highlight your qualities, apart from not appearing arrogant, you should avoid constantly talking about yourself. Women like men who are active listeners and not those who exalt themselves.

2. How to seduce a woman

To captivate a woman you just have to bet on your true genuine personality and move forward slowly, but also without pause.
Make her feel very comfortable with you in all areas, listening to her, fixing your gaze in her eyes and complimenting her when it seems appropriate. Falling in love with her will be possible when empathy and respect are enveloping them, there she will begin to feel attracted to you.

3. Wear fancy clothes

If you choose the right clothes to introduce yourself to your date, it will not take long to see how she felt dazzled, from hair to the tips of her shoes, by your manly elegance. Picking up a girl starts with your personal appearance and follows in the kind and captivating attitude you have towards her.

4. What to say to attract her

To interest a woman has a lot to do, above all, knowing how to listen. It is essential, but then you should take advantage of an informal chat to attach some loving phrases that will speak well of you, if they are not too far-fetched or too listened to over time.

Originality, healthy mischief and the way you are going to say them, is what will go down wonderfully and will attract a woman that you already have in your sights.

5. Take care of your personal appearance
You are going to need to feel confident about your appearance and leave no doubt about yourself, about how you will be presenting yourself to woo the girl you like.
Of course, a good bath is essential, then a fragrance on the skin that does not stun the senses, but rather that gently intoxicates it and finally, a shoe according to your clothing, neatly cared for. Your hair and how you fix it will also play a role as an infallible weapon of seduction

6. Do not rush to show yourself as a friend
When you start dating her, you won't want to show yourself like a simple friend would. You have to direct yourself with a plan that leads you to fall in love with her.

Quite simply, she will want you to look at her, talk to her and treat her absolutely like someone trying to seduce her, with bold phrases or conversations, although always within a respectful limit.

7. Respect punctuality in your appointments
An especially difficult woman will not tolerate you leaving her in a sit-in waiting for you. While it is true that anyone can be delayed, do not think that this way you will be able to conquer that person, much more if you have done it more than once.

Being and showing yourself pleasant will have to do with attending your outings with her in a timely manner, that will give you extra credit for you to advance and appear before her eyes as a true gentleman.

8. Act without invading their expectations
There are different ways for humans to fall in love with a girl that attracts them a lot. The clear example of overwhelming to lose indicates that, if you are thinking of obtaining success by running over her expectations with respect to you, you are putting the worst obstacle for her to decide for herself and freely.

The unwanted pressures will not bring you to fruition ... and much less with a complicated girl!

9. You must be yourself

Nothing worse than pretending to be someone else. Much less trying to be the Man She is looking for. Lies are impossible to sustain for long. In the end, you don't want a person to fall in love with a non-existent being.

10. Be patient, don't rush things

When you get that woman longed for by your heart to accept your first date, you must have perseverance and above all patience, so as not to fall overboard of your excessive impulses. You have to bear in mind that, in every process, in this case of conquest, you have to respect the steps to follow, so that everything goes with the best results. The greatest successes ... were in the hands of patience!

11. Mention clever phrases that move her

Words spoken with intelligence and enthusiasm can be a delight to the person in question. A romantic approach with subliminal and psychological phrases can get you much more than you really want when it comes to flirting her.

The ways to get that woman's attention can have results you never imagined for your own happiness and that of your future partner.

12. Stand out like no other with a special lotion

As most of us know, on the market today there are substances that increase male libido, components of particular lotions.

It is very important that you try one of them. Fragrances of all kinds can captivate that girl in a crazy way, in your favor. Choose the scent that you know she may like, after informal and informative talks.

To attract them, and make them feel comfortable with you, I recommend that you use perfumes with pheromones for men

13. Be sure of yourself and show it

Perhaps you should look within and recognize your most remarkable qualities. Confidently highlight all those virtues you possess without being presumptuous, far from it. Your behavior must flow without colliding or exceeding the normal limits so as not to play against your interest, which is to charm your desired girl.

14. Be romantic, but not cloying

Never try to conquer the person who is breaking your heart with kitsch or phrases that you may regret tomorrow.

Do not try to overshadow your true personality, because if you try to pretend someone you are not, sooner or later they will find out, and you will not have gotten anything positive from all the time you invested in her. Capturing her attention and making her fall in love always arises from being authentic. There is no other positive way.

15. Show him the things you share

The more he feels that he shares things in common with you, the better he will feel around you. Always handle conversations, but let the necessary spread by manifesting what makes him happy in life, in this way he will subconsciously associate you with positive events.

You are always trying to find out more about your aspirations in life, what makes you happy, if you don't feel comfortable talking about something, change the subject. You can talk about negative topics later, now is the time for me to associate you with positive topics.

16. Keeping the mystery

It is healthy that you maintain a certain air of mystery, so you will make her miss you, and need you. If you are constantly in his personal space, he may get bored of you. So you must manage a balance. Don't be too intense, but don't stray that far either. I know! It sounds a bit complex, as complex as women are.

Many people ask me: how to manipulate a woman ?, and the truth is that each woman is a world, so you have to discover her, she probably does not like that you are aware of her at all times. Or it could also be that type of girl who wants you to constantly write or call. As time goes by, you will discover the actions that he expects of you.

17. Talk in occasional appointments and get to know her

It is highly recommended that you use those occasional long talks to learn about their personal tastes, needs, and ambitions. Sometimes there are "talks" but not dialogues, and this is the first point where a pretended conquest can succumb.

It is extremely necessary that you know what kind of music he likes, if he likes to dance and if he has favorite literary authors. From then on, communication deepens.

18. Cautiously inquire about her love past

Of course, without being insidious with the questions and without questioning how much she wants to tell you, but make it clear that everything she tells you will give you an overview, for your possible and future relationship. Sometimes informal talks collect the best data.

19. Subtly find out their current marital status

It may happen that the girl shows herself as distant from your interests for a simple and complex reason at the same time, such as the fact that she remains married to another person and maintains a formal and distant posture in the eyes of others.

This does not mean that, for that reason, you cannot get to have a formal relationship with her, despite the social obstacles. You will be in charge of searching for the truth.

20. Find your personal strategy in these ideas

The ideas that I am expressing here, I want you to take them as basic rules to reach your heart.

Some will seem good to you, others better, the issue is that you have a strategic plan that allows you to achieve with the help of this blog and its advice, the essentials to get closer to that woman who has you enraptured with love.

21. Get him used to you

This tip is almost fundamental, I would tell you. A follow-up by chat, phone or by any means that seems appropriate, will work in your favor. Be consistent and stay in constant communication with that person.

She will feel contained by you and will want to keep hearing your voice constantly. It is then when the so-called accustoming or "abstinence" occurs and you will already be reflected in their thoughts permanently, with which you will have half the battle won.

22. Get to know your relatives again

A very important detail in a man who wants to flirt with a woman is to get closer to his closest family or his closest friends. Connect with respect and cordiality, get involved in the dialogues and participate with interest in comments or events that are being touched on in occasional talks.

By empathizing with the relatives of the young woman in question, you will have gained part of her heart.

23. Surprise her with minimal details

Fill her with tenderness by asking her, for example, if her sick pet got better or if the headache she had the night before has gone away. No gift will bring you closer to her than considering her and taking her into account in special and personal situations.

24. Do not rush the topic of intimacy: Wait!

Do not pressure or force situations that have to do with intimacy. She will take her time to re-categorize you, she will keep in mind some things she experienced, which were disastrous and she will not want to repeat similar experiences. If you have achieved a rapprochement, don't spoil it all… Wait!

25. Avoid talking about sex on first dates.

Here we reinforce the idea of the previous tip. If you are going to talk about sex, not on the first or on the second date and if it comes up on the third, it is because it happened naturally and not because you provoked it. Do not spoil the path sown with a stone trodden out of time.

26. Organize outings creatively

When you invite her for a walk, organize an outing that she likes and is excited about. Ask her where she would like to go and if it is within your means, take her to that fun and picturesque place that she will never forget!

27. Rough male vs sensitive male

It depends on the woman, she will show more interest in one type of man, or another. Who attracts more attention ?, the manly, or the sensitive ?. It depends!.

To know it you must know her well, and know exactly what she is looking for, good communication will always be basic to seduce a woman. If you have any questions, you can ask him about the previous boyfriends, what they worked on, studied, what their hobbies were, and with that information you will know what initially catches his attention.

Remember that you should never change, you will only use this information in an informative way, think about what you have in common with your "ex" and bring it up. Ask him about his favorite movie, singer, about his relationship with his parents. Find the right time to ask. You will be surprised at how much you will learn from her.

When you know if you like manly males, more than sensitive ones, or vice versa, use that information to praise those qualities that you have and fit your needs.

28. Avoid drinking too much if you are with her

It will not be pleasant for the girl who fell in love to see you arrive on a date almost drunk or smelling of cigarettes.

Being delicate in that regard will prevent her from rejecting you when you see you like this. There are few men who, to give themselves courage when facing a reluctant woman, turn to drink to "reinforce" their courage. Keep this in mind when going to meet him.

29. Humor as a tool

With all the good energy and a big smile, the world is conquered ... and how much more a girl who has you full of love. Make that woman laugh until you are tired and walk towards the happiness of her hand, laughter is healing and if it comes from you, it is absolutely sublime.

For a man in love there are no possible obstacles to reach his wife, no matter how complicated the relationship that lies ahead may be. Daring is the mechanism that will allow you to achieve what you daydream about, what you want intensely. Nothing equals the courage you show trying to hold that woman surrendered in your arms... It's worth a try!

Mistakes you should not make in bed.

When it comes to the needs of women in bed, some men make a number of mistakes that they could avoid. But what are these mistakes? We answer this question in the following lines:

1. Start sex in the bedroom

While men turn on at the speed of light, in the case of women, this is not exactly the case. For many women, feeling secure in the relationship and confident with the person next to them is what is really going to make the sexual encounter great.

That is why it is necessary to work on sex outside the room, with kisses, hugs, fun moments ... A simple hug may be more important than many think, because 30 seconds of hug stimulate oxytocin, a hormone that creates connection and trust with the other person. Something that will have a positive impact on intimate moments.

2. Thinking you know what he wants

Each person is different and, in terms of sexual tastes, not everyone enjoys the same things. For example, there are people who like unconventional situations and there are people with more classic sexual tastes. Therefore, it is important that there is communication and do not be afraid to ask what the other person likes in order to meet their expectations.

3. Overdoing it with rough sex

And of course, regarding the intensity of sex there are also different tastes and opinions. Not bad at all a little intensity when it is consensual. But many women agree when trust and affection prevail. So once the sexual act is over, you need to consider her needs. A loving hug is a good alternative.

4. Not treating the clitoris well

Women enjoy clitoral stimulation and this is something every man knows. So the clitoris should never be forgotten. However, at the same time, you have to know how to play this key, and it's not about scratching or rubbing, but about getting it right. Remember that the clitoris is extremely sensitive, so touching too hard when it's not the right time can be painful.

5. Focusing on the breasts and genitals too quickly

When it comes to stimulating a woman, it is necessary to do it gradually. The skin is full of nerve endings and knowing how to touch it can be very effective in preparing other people to take action. That the preliminaries are important is not a myth but is a reality and therefore must be paid attention so that the woman fully enjoys it.

6. Ignore mental stimulation

When we talk about foreplay, many people have physical stimulation in mind. However, the mental aspect is very important so that the level of arousal increases. While the stimulation of men is almost instantaneous and what they see is enough for them, women are especially turned on by their fantasies and their expectations.

7. Forget about creativity

Many couples, when they have been long, complain of monotony. And it is that being creative is one of the best ways to keep the flame of passion in life. Especially when the relationship has stabilized, it is necessary to use resources that allow the flame not to go out. What if you play naked twister or do a bodypainting session?

8. Pay attention to the conclusion

For many women, one of the most important parts of having sex is how it ends. Once a man reaches orgasm he can do two things. Have a cold ending and rest or melt into a hug with the other person for a relatively long period of time to show affection. Being a cold and unemotional man influences sexual satisfaction.

Dirty things to say to a girl to get her wet with

Why is dirty talk so effective?

We all know how good it is to activate people. Saying the right things can lead someone who is not in the mood to dribble. But you need to know what dirty things to say to a girl will really work.

You must be descriptive. The reason dirty talk is so sexy is because it takes people to an extremely specific place on their mind. They imagine the things you are talking about and the memories of how those things feel is what makes their body irritated and ready to go.

All the dirty things to tell a girl they want her bad

If you are looking for a way to make your woman horny as hell, we have what you need. These are all dirty things to say to a girl that she will get wet and beg her to satisfy her.

1 "I want you to take me right now."

2 "I want my face between your legs."

3 "I can't stop thinking about how good you feel."

4 "I wish my hands were combing through your hair, pulling it, making you moan with pleasure."

5 "The sounds you made the last time we were in bed made me so weak."

6 "Just thinking about your nude drives me crazy."

7 "I just can't control myself when I think about defeating you."

8 "Can't you tell how horny you are? Make me just be you?"

9 "I've been thinking about being inside you all day."

10 "I love your taste"

11 "My hands, running down your body. I need it."

12 "Tonight, I want you to be in charge."

13 "Whatever you want me to do to you, I'll do it."

14 "The idea that I give you on the counter will not leave me."

15 "I want to undress you and feel your body up and down."

16 "Let me make you feel better than you ever have before."

17 "I want my tongue on your clit, making you moan for hours."

18 "Tonight, I'm yours. Tell me what you want."

19 "The way you feel below me is addictive. I can't get enough."

20 "I need to be careful around you. I just can't think straight."

21 "I'm going to turn you over and you're going to take it."

22 "I want you to take control right now."

23 "I can't help but complain when I'm in your mouth."

24 "I want to make you scream with pleasure tonight."

25 "I want to be so into you."

26 "I've never been this tough before."

27 "You're so tight, I can't take it."

28 "Hmm, I could do this all night."

29 "Your body in mine is what I long for."

30 "I want to bring you down for hours."

TIPS TO MAKE YOUR DIRTY TALK EVEN MORE POWERFUL

These phrases may seem perfectly useful, but only if you know how and when to use them. Here are some tips to get the most out of talking dirty with your girl.

1 Say something really bad in public. Nothing is sexier than a really intimate and naughty man in a public setting. Obviously, you want to shut up and make sure no one else can hear you. But if you do this right, it will be a big change for her. Just whisper what you want to say low into her ear and watch her squirm.

2 Send it by text. If you're not together, take the opportunity to text her something very dirty. Not only will you make her feel horny while you are away from you, but it will also increase the anticipation for a good time later.

This can also give you an opportunity to practice sexting. There's nothing better than getting really turned on by a good dirty texting conversation.

3 Give her a slow, romantic kiss, and end it by whispering in her ear. This is extremely effective due to the parallels. A really deep and romantic kiss will already turn her on and then she will say something very dirty when she is expecting something sweet.

The surprise and your words specifically will make her feel wet for you. After doing this, you can take things to the bedroom!

4 Know what he likes. If you know what your girl likes, you can better tailor what she says. The dirty things to say to a girl who works best are always the ones that will pique her the most interest.

If you know that your girl loves it when you fall in love with her, then focus on that. Talk about how much you love it and how much you wish you could have her right there. You'll start to imagine this and you'll be hot in no time.

5 Just say what feels natural. Don't try to say a lot of these things if they sound strange and awkward coming out of your mouth. That will basically ruin the moment.

If you are new to this, start slowly. Start with simple sentences that make sense. "I love you so bad" is a perfect place to start. You can also see how much your partner is reacting and continue down a path that you are responding well to.

Knowing what dirty things to say to a girl that turns her on will be helpful for many reasons. Next time you want it to be yours in the bedroom, try some of these.

Woman who are good in bed do these things

To be honest, we must admit that there are many girls who have no idea how to be a ten under the sheets. An expert on the subject details what the 'cracks' of sex do

Much is written about what they must do in bed to please women. It is normal that sex articles tend to be focused on the male sector: most have no idea how to treat a female under the sheets (or outside of bed, but that is another issue). From this section we want to be egalitarian, so today we will dedicate a topic to what the ladies have to do in terms of sexual relations. Also, to be totally fair, we must recognize that there are many girls who have no idea how to be a ten in bed. The reasons for your malpractice are different from theirs. As a general rule, they do not know how to act, and they know but they are self-conscious for dozens of reasons.

One of the most powerful is the fear they have when they think that if they behave wildly horizontally, their beloved will stop seeing them with the eyes of a "future wife" and only as a "lover".

Women considered good in bed do not cut themselves when taking the first step. Many desire it strongly, they insinuate themselves, but they fail to act.

"They try not to be the 'whore' or 'bitch' girl because they want to take them home to meet their parents. But they forget that this 'bitch' girl (in bed) is the one who will take away their place in the relationship" , says the expert, who recommends that all women behave with their loved one (or that being they have just met) as they really feel, without falling into stupid and outdated prejudices.

Sex, in all its variables, is made to be enjoyed, as a couple or alone. In the first case, even more so, that is why they (and they) must let go (always with health first) when they are together. Dedicated to them, Tracey exposes the eight things that every woman who is considered "good in bed" does. Attentive:

1 They take the initiative.

"She never takes the first step" or "I always have to be the one to initiate the sexual relationship" are the main male complaints in this intimate field. Tracey is clear: if you always let him be the one to start, bad. Women considered good in bed do not cut themselves when they start a relationship. Many want it strongly, they insinuate themselves, but they fail to act. Enough already, if you want, let him know. They love it.

2 They have no prejudices.

Often happens. He proposes something new in bed and she replies with a resounding NO! intrinsically linked to the thought "I always knew hc was weird." Woman, free yourself. Maybe you even like it. We are obviously referring to common propositions. Everyone has somewhat strange fantasies or predilections. The subject of the same considers them "peculiarities", while his partner may see them as "perverted". It has always been said that you can see if someone is good or bad in bed depending on how much or how little they like to give and receive oral sex "If your partner suggests you do something that you have never considered, think will this make me harm to me (or him or a third party) physically or emotionally? If the answer is no, what are you waiting for? Open minded women are what men consider cracks in bed."

3 They are not afraid to say 'NO'

Related to the previous point, you do not always have to say yes. Not much less. Women who say yes to every request for the sole purpose of pleasing their partner are anything but sexy. The sexologist relates that once a man came to her consultation and told her that he had completely lost his desire for his girlfriend because everything he proposed was accepted and followed by her. "It was too evident that there was no enjoyment on both sides," says the expert. The boy in question alleged that his partner was watching him carefully to see if he was enjoying himself, completely forgetting about his own pleasure. "Actually, he had no idea what she liked, because he never let her know."

Occasionally you must please the couple by doing things that they like, but also ask. "Sexual honesty is essential."

4 They like to try new things.

"I have hundreds of emails on this topic: 'Why don't you want to watch porn with me / let me shave your sex / keep my shoes on during intercourse / look in a mirror / masturbate for me / go out without underwear?' What is basically extracted from all these issues is the rejection of some women for doing things that they have never seen or done before. "

The matter is truly clear: imagine that you always have a hamburger for dinner, which you love but ... it ends up getting you tired after a while. Well, the same thing happens with relationships: sleeping with the same person is like having the same food over and over again. That is why you must innovate from time to time.

5 They praise the penis.

Men are not only concerned with the size of their penis: they are also concerned with how long it stays hard and what it looks like (whether it is pretty or ugly). Those who are good in bed assiduously pay attention to their partner's penis: they look at it, talk to it (within limits), praise it ('oh, how big and hard') ... and they love it.

6 They are exceptionally good at oral sex It has always been said (and we fully agree) that you can tell if someone is good or bad in bed based on how much or how little they enjoy giving and receiving oral sex.

If your partner suggests you do something that you have never considered, think, will it hurt me? If the answer is negative, what are you waiting for? Think about it: there is nothing more intimate than letting the other person put their mouth on your genitals, or vice versa. Much more personal than standard intercourse. "Oral sex is the most personal side of relationships and doing it (and receiving it) means that you are not scrupulous and accept that sex is chaotic and sweaty."

All men want to be the best that has passed through the sheets of their current partner. A bit out of ego and a bit out of love for the other person, because there is nothing more beautiful than making someone you love to enjoy. As we said at the beginning of the topic, they often do not do it well because they simply do not know. That is why it is good that she gives directions, and only those who are good, sexually speaking, do. [10 things they want to try in bed and do not tell you] "He wants instructions on how to please you, but he doesn't want to ask for fear of sounding silly," says Tracey. You can be more subtle: When he does something, you like exactly how you like it, let him know with a "keep doing exactly that."

8 They make noise (but not too much)

Have you ever had sex with someone who was super quiet and did not make a sound? We do, and it's pretty unnerving. It looks like you are with a dead man or a robot. Equally disturbing are those individuals who do not stop talking or moaning very loudly. There is a point in between that is fair, and the same that the 'cracks of sex' dominate perfectly. Go ahead! Sex is life, do not be told otherwise.

Most effective techniques for female orgasm

Despite the immense advances that have been made -after years of struggle- to achieve full independence from women, in certain domains the male domination persists; and for example, topics such as female self-satisfaction continue to feel taboo topics.
Together with the University of Indiana and the Kinsey Institute, both in the United States, they carried out a huge study to learn more about this displaced issue. The idea: to share the techniques, until now secret, with which women manage to increase sexual pleasure.
between 20 and 30 percent of heterosexual women never achieve orgasm during their sexual encounters. Other studies go as far as raising that figure to 50 percent. And the majority (68%, according to recent research) continue to fake the climax in front of their partners, even knowing that there is not the solution.
"The taboo that makes people uncomfortable with female anatomy is the same one that has kept female pleasure a secret for far too long. That is the taboo we want to get rid of. We believe that people are prepared for an honest and clear look at the details that make the difference. "
Less than 20% of women reach orgasm through penetration.
This first phase of the study has focused on the clitoris - that organ of the woman's body intended solely for pleasure. In fact, according to Kim, women have four times more orgasms with stimulation than with penetration.

"Only 17% of women have a penetrative orgasm. 73% of women surveyed said that stimulation of the clitoris during penetration led to better orgasms." Let's not forget that the stimulation of 8,000 nerve endings in the clitoris causes greater pleasure with minimal effort.

The 10 techniques have received different names, chosen by the women surveyed: "In sex we have a limited vocabulary, something that does not help, for example, it has come to terms such as "giving clues", which consists of passing the fingers, but only occasionally giving pleasure. "Rhythm", an almost musical movement, looped. And the most desired: "Multiple", for her multiple orgasms. Women have created these names and are finally able to express what they want to try.

Breaking down the 10 techniques

1- Bordering Edging

It is a simple principle: it is about stimulating the sensitive regions little by little and when the woman is about to reach orgasm (here is the difficult part), lower the intensity of the stimulation or stop completely. You can repeat the process several times. This causes the accumulation of tension to increase more and more. The result? A much more intense orgasm. 65.5% of the women surveyed say it worked for them.

2- Hinting

With this technique, the purpose is to find a tender point (such as the clitoris), but not go directly to it. The idea is to feel the ground and go around that spot, touching it only occasionally. This would be a kind of heating and then start stimulating these regions with greater intensity. 71% of those surveyed say it works, experts say.

3- Consistency

Many women assured that at the moment when orgasm is approaching, a good procedure is to follow exactly the same rhythm that initially generated the beginning of orgasm. If you speed up or slow down the rhythm, as well as if you increase or decrease the intensity, the orgasm can be much less, or it can even be lost.

4- Surprise

Seven out of ten women who participated in the study say that it is much better when stimulation has its changes. The idea is not to stay in the monotony of the sexual act or masturbation and to play with the changes of intensity and time intervals. What you should do is not generate a too repetitive pattern. Here, creativity plays an especially important role.

5- Multiple

Surely you have heard of this type of climax sometime. 47% of the study participants claim to have had multiple orgasms at some time. The common mistake here is to continue with the exact same type of stimulation that led to the woman having her first orgasm. After the climax, certain parts are sensitive, so if you do the same, it can hurt. The idea is to vary the movements.

6- Accenting

Every woman has different tender points around the clitoris. The secret here is to emphasize stimulation in those parts that generate the greatest sensation of pleasure. This, without neglecting the other areas, which must also be stimulated, although with less intensity.

7- Framing

This is a series of techniques that does not lie so much in the physical part, but in the psychological side during the sexual act. Distracting thoughts can be fatal to an orgasm. How to avoid them? For example, it is mentioned that many women surveyed affirm that the fact of thinking about reaching the climax has taken them away from it. The ideal is not to get carried away by worries and insecurities and just enjoy the act.

8- By layers

The clitoris is an extremely sensitive organ. This is why stimulating it directly is not such a good idea. The idea of this technique is to gradually accentuate the layers of skin that surround the clitoris, so that in this way the woman accumulates sexual tension, but gradually.

9- Rhythm

Creating certain patterns and using rhythm in stimulation can be a great advantage. Like playing an instrument, either through masturbation or penetration, it is important to put a kind of metronome to the movements. Ideally, this rhythm is not always the same, but changes and modifies as the sexual act progresses.

10- Staging

OMGYes identified certain stages of female sexual arousal: desire building, prewarming, increasing arousal, approaching climax, orgasm, and finally multiple orgasm. Each stage varies from woman to woman and what may be pleasant at one time can also be uncomfortable at another; it all depends on the circumstance.

In the future, those responsible for OMGYes will seek to approach other areas of sexual pleasure, such as internal stimulation, penetration angles, squirting (or female ejaculation), breathing, oral sex, pleasure during pregnancy and postpartum, sex during menopause. And integrate experiences of LGTBI people.

Tricks for women to agree to oral sex.

Not all women are willing to do it, that is why you need to make her talk about her fears and make her feel more comfortable, at first it will seem strange to have this conversation but talking about intimate matters will help them develop more trust and intimacy, although she objects to the idea. If you feel uncomfortable talking about it, she will notice and she will feel uncomfortable too, being close to your wife will help you stay one step ahead.

Helpful Wisdom: Women are not so fond of oral sex. A Canadian study revealed that only 28% of the girls surveyed indicated that performing oral sex "was very pleasant." Just over half said it was "somewhat pleasant" and 17% said they had not enjoyed it at all. - Men´s Health

1.- Honesty. Talk openly about the subject, tell her what you want, but in the following way: Find out what she likes, what turns her on and what gives her pleasure, after this, talk about what gives you pleasure. Make your conversation intimate and two-way, choose the right moment, without interruptions. Do not pressure her, just start by confiding in her the things you like best in sex. Offer your wife or girlfriend a conversation of respect, love, and trust, thus making her more open.

2.- Do not press. It is possible that he does not speak much of the subject and that he says no, let him speak so much or little what he says. You have already expressed your wishes and she will be aware of what you like, so do not pressure her, even in a subtle way. The worst thing you could do is pressure or force her.

3.- Understand it. Consider the reason why she might not want to do it, she is in a vulnerable position, she also might feel nauseous and choking. She could cause you discomfort, do not dismiss her concerns or focus only on your desires.

4.- Give her the best oral sex of her life. Become an expert in doing oral sex, after the dialogue try to become an expert in how to do oral sex to a woman, she will be very satisfied and may pretend to want to return the favor.

5.- Stay desirable. Stay clean, groomed, and clean, give him no reason to hesitate if you have bathed.

6.- Do not set expectations. Your wife is not a porn actress, adult film actresses are professionals and experts in such activities, something that your wife or partner is not.

7.- Give him control. If you are going to place your hand on her head, do it gently, just to hold her hair so she does not interrupt, do it gently and allow her to feel comfortable.

8.- Play around. Once they have discussed it, she plays by putting a condom in her mouth, as if to imply that you want her to try to put it on with her lips. Put on whipped cream or some other edible substance with a pleasant taste, this will encourage her to continue with the game and to please you.

How to move your tongue when giving your girl oral sex

Oral sex is the old practice of stimulating your girl with your wet, long, and hot tongue, many think that to do this you do not need tricks or tips, they are wrong that is why their women leave them or they do not reach orgasm in their relationships.
Oral sex is the game prior to a good time of wild sex that we all know, that is, it sets things right for a pleasant penetration. But it's better that you don't throw yourself into your girl's vagina like a dog when they throw a piece of meat at her, you have to be tactful and have very good movements.
First you must find the clitoris you can find it in the labia minora, and it is like a small fleshy prominent part, like the rubber of a pencil. Since you found that pleasant part of the woman, now if to put your language to work.

Circles. The one that everyone applies, and which has incredibly good results. Move your tongue in circles gently passing it through the vagina, first from left to right and after a while from right to left. You will know that you are doing well with your girl's movements and contractions. On the contrary, if you feel a hit, better leave it and watch a movie.

Cone tongue. You can also make it rigid, - we are talking about the tongue - not so firm, in the shape of a cone, perform fast and slow movements from top to bottom and from left to right or hitting the clitoris a little with it.

her lips. Another good technique of how to move your tongue when giving oral sex to your girl is to suck her clitoris gently, add to that slight pressure of lips the stimulation with the tongue.

Cow lick. There are girls and boys who like to extend their tongues and who lick like ice cream or a cow lick because with this you not only cover the clitoris but also other parts of the vagina. They can start gently and tenderly until they exert a little more pressure.

The combination. Try moving your tongue over the clitoris so lightly that you barely touch it, then alternately wet your lips and do the same. Every so often, go back a little and simply breathe on the area, your breath will pink her body and make her feel a very pleasant tingle. With this you will not know if it is coming or going, literally.

Penetration. For a moment she leaves the clitoris alone for a moment, and better insert it as deep as you can inside her vagina in a single throw. She is going to love this because she feels so good, because her tongue is fine and strong, and she can move while she is still inside her.

If you still wondered how to move your tongue when giving oral sex to your girl, now you know. With these movements your girlfriend will not have eyes for another guy and her orgasms will be guaranteed. Good luck killer! or Licker?

7 positions for oral sex, prepare your tongue.

The mythical and always reliable 69:
Here both receive and give pleasure at the same time and either you love her, or you hate her. It is more fun than normal oral sex.

Doggylingus:
Orgasmic posture prior to intercourse that does not have to play any specific role. This combines oral sex with masturbation is simple and comfortable. As I have said before, it allows multiple stimuli, for both men and women.

Submissive fellatio:
A classic and exciting position for men, this is also exclusively for the pleasure of the male sex. She on her knees and you standing in front of her recommended for couples who know each other and know what and how to play. The look of love is born from this position.

Deep oral:
Exclusive to women and more if you are one of those who have a hard time reaching orgasm via intercourse. In this lying on the bed or on some flat surface both legs are raised and expose the vagina. So, the man's wet tongue goes deeper as he pats your thighs and butt.

Lateral oral:
Here both of you lying on the bed turn on your side and face each other. She gets down until she has his penis close to her face and gives him her. The purpose of this position is that your knees do not suffer from a cramp in the neck.

She standing:
This is something rare, but you will make her scream with pleasure (of course, as long as you fight with the language). Place her in front of a mirror, your kneeling in front of her and then put your tongue on her vulva.

The romantic:

Equally directed to them, here you can use the edge of any surface, the kitchen table, the dining room table, the washing machine, a desk etc. She is sitting on the surface resting her heels on the edge of it, you can start to work, she will feel less exposed, super excited and finally she can hug her to make her feel more united and give her more complicity.

Ready, do you already have them? Well, they hope to take advantage of them and run to practice each of these positions to give the best oral sex, surely, they will be pleased and willing to repeat it over and over and over and over again.

Things women hate about oral sex.

There are many reasons, some things make women hate giving their boys oral sex. Here are some of the things women hate about doing oral sex on their partners. Pay close attention, knowing it can help you make the moment less uncomfortable and more pleasant.

1.- That you try to convince them. Women hate, the more you try to convince them to suck you off, be so insistent. She is not going to force you to make her cunnilingus, better be smarter and she tries to persuade her without being too insistent. Try with your tongue on her clitoris and her vagina, maybe later you will be rewarded for your good work.

2.- Force her head. Perhaps your desires will drive you to make disturbing movements, like push your girl's head towards you while she does oral sex, if she was not very convinced, be sure that she will not spoil you again. Trying to make her eat your whole package will make her choke on it or make her want to vomit.

3.- Not being able to breathe. One of the most uncomfortable things for a woman to have your package in her mouth is not being able to breathe well, so what you can do for her benefit is to allow her to take breaks.

4.- The hairs. The sex is rich, but the hairs are somewhat uncomfortable, especially if a hair is left in her mouth or in her throat. You would not like it, definitely not her.

5.- The smells. An uncomfortable moment for a woman who finally dared to give you oral sex is that you have poor hygiene, try to wash your thing well and that your balls are not smelling of sweat, definitely the first thing they perceive when doing it with their mouth are the smells.
6.- That there is no reciprocity.
Not only does it mean that you will do cunnilingus later, it means that you will do it very well, many girls expect reciprocity, so try to give it quality. Worry that she enjoys it too.

7.- Their jaw hurts.
Moderate yourself, what would you feel if you had your jaw open for a long time? Obviously, you would get tired. Let your girl alternate or her jaws will go numb.

8.- Semen surprise.
Depending on your diet, the taste of semen changes, your girl may or may not like the taste of your honey. She tries to warn him before coming into her mouth and above all, she respects her decision.

9.- They do not enjoy.
She alternates with kisses and caresses, plays with her breasts, or does 69, the point is that she does not lose excitement either.

10.- Hurt you.
Many women may be concerned about hurting you with their teeth, so they try to avoid giving you oral sex.

How to talk to my partner to have a threesome?

If you are reading this, you probably want to have a threesome, but your partner probably does not agree to the idea easily. Well, there are several things that you must consider and which you must argue and with them give security to your partner, so that he ends up accepting.

I will start by giving some tips that you should consider before talking to your partner about the subject:

Making a threesome is not easy, it leads to a complete disorder of feelings and moral judgments, before doing it, try to have a very mature and safe relationship. Normally couples do not accept having threesomes due to insecurity; They think of possibilities that they cannot control, such as: That their partner plans to meet the other person again to have secret sex, or that the person invited to the threesome likes their partner more than themselves; or that the person invited to the threesome is better than them in bed.

Read, learn, and watch porn videos that give you a better idea of how to have a threesome. Pleasing your partner many times is not so easy, now imagine pleasing two people at the same time; basically, you must perform for two; reading, learning, and watching videos will give you many ideas and techniques that you can take advantage of.

Know very well what your threesome partners like, talk to them and ask them, so you will have an advantage and you will not bore either of them.

Do not propose a threesome to your partner with an ex-girlfriend or person that you like sentimentally.

If your partner is a heterosexual woman:
She will not accept a threesome with another woman, if you do not know how to convince her or at least make her curious about what it would be like to have sex with a woman. It is easier for her to agree to have a threesome with a man, so you must be willing to have sex with one, make sure that man is bisexual. And if you are not willing to have sex with a man, she will probably not accept, for the simple reason that her partner is not going to enjoy it, creating a heavy atmosphere and post-sex arguments.

If your partner is a bisexual woman:

It is much easier for her to agree to have sex with a woman or a man, it is scientifically proven that bisexual people tend to be a little more promiscuous than heterosexual or homosexual people, which is an advantage in these cases. Ask your partner, which would please him more, have sex with a man or a woman, knowing this, you have a guideline to find a sexual partner.

If your partner is a lesbian woman:
Do not propose to do a threesome with a man unless she has mentioned that curiosity before and you, as a woman partner, also want to experience it. Get a delicate partner, if she decides that he is a man, as a brusque man, he probably creates some kind of phobia and pain in you. If he is a woman, try to know the tastes of your partner, even propose to find it between the two of you.

If your partner is a heterosexual man:
He will not accept to have a threesome with a man, look for a woman with different qualities or beauty or contrast to yours, who obviously likes him, so you will create a more aphrodisiac and fantastic environment, if he is looking for a partner very similar to you, he will prefer to be more focused on you and they will bore the partner.

If your partner is a bisexual man:
It is extremely easy for him to agree to have a threesome with you, I do not know that he proposes it, they look for a partner together, and argue the sentimental love that they feel for each other, propose some rules, but not obligations, because as bisexual couples tend to being more promiscuous, sexual intercourse may repeat itself. Do not make threesomes starting a relationship, it will surely end after this experience.

If your partner is a homosexual man:
Homosexual couples tend to be very possessive, try to propose the threesome with great delicacy and without obfuscating the feelings of your partner, as this proposition can lead to misunderstandings: "I don't please him in bed." Find a man you do not know and use a lot of protection. Remember that AIDS, it is much easier to be acquired by anal penetration.

Protection must be important:
Remember the safe sex protocol: oral, vagina, then anal; If they violate this order, they run the risk of contagion of disease and alteration in ph. Use condoms, I recommend the use of female condoms in threesomes of one man, two women and the use of male condoms in threesomes: three men; and threesomes of one woman and two men. In lesbian threesomes, a lot of oral and vaginal hygiene and please, hygiene in your hands.
The use of sex toys will facilitate the orgasm of your sexual partners and will help you to please one, while enjoying the other.
To convince your partner you can:
Watch threesome porn videos with hers. And argue because it would be pleasant for him / her, along with things that you like.
Suggest going to swinger bars.
Download articles that discuss the emotional benefits that a threesome brings to a couple's relationship.
Find the right moment to do it, try to excite him / her when you propose and fantasize about it.

Seek help from a psychologist or sexologist.

Create controversy about it in your social group and give excellent contributions, to create curiosity in your partner and know their point of view.
I hope that after reading this article you have the best threesome of your life, with your partner and safely.

Some tips to enjoy it.

Once you have found a way to do a threesome, don't forget the following:

Choose your candidates well.
It is not enough to have thought whether the chosen person will be a friend or a stranger. It is important that there is attraction and that there is a good feeling. And that includes that there are similar tastes or preferences in bed, so that no one is surprised.

Security before everything
For everyone is good, do not be shy about asking the other people involved if they have any possible sexually transmitted diseases that you should be aware of. And above all, use protection.

Spread your attention.
In order to do a threesome and make it satisfactory for everyone, this should be a balanced activity and you should try to focus your attention on everyone involved equally. If you do it with your partner, this will prevent possible jealousy or reproach for having paid more attention to the third person.

Painless anal sex

What is anal sex?
Anal sex is the direct sexual stimulation of the anus and nearby areas. Apart from penetration, oral and manual stimulation is considered.

Why do couples have anal sex?
The anus is a powerful erogenous zone capable of providing a great amount of pleasure to both men and women. Although the man, more than the woman, since his g-spot, is in this part.

Why is anal sex painful?
The fact that it is considered a painful practice is because to enjoy anal penetration requires patience, consideration, and large amounts of lubricant. The ideal is to lick, suck or caress, so said pain will not exist.

Furthermore, we must bear in mind that the anus is a sphincter, that is, a "closure" in this case of the intestine that is designed to let out, to expel. So, if the body feels that something wants to enter through the anus, the body will immediately choose to close it with more force.
Add to the above, the fact of not having its own lubrication, the important thing about lubrication is that there is no friction. When there is dry friction, it not only hurts but it burns, which is dangerous, as the skin can tear and even bleed.

What to do, so that this practice is not painful?
The main thing to enjoy this game is to start small. I in my mind argue some steps from my experience, which may be useful to you.

Relax the sphincter.

For the sphincter to relax and open, the ideal would be to start stimulating it orally since the tongue is soft, smooth, and moist. You can lick, suck, kiss, or bite gently, these provide great pleasure and get used to the area to contact.

Stimulate manually.

For the record, we have not yet introduced anything anywhere, we just caress and massage, with lubricant if possible; If you do not have lubricant, heterosexual and lesbian couples can use vaginal lubrication, while gay couples can use saliva. (Some gay men recommend the use of petroleum jelly instead of lubricant.)
While we massage the area gently, there can (and should) be kisses, caresses, genital masturbation, words, back massages, soft slaps on the buttocks ... who knows, it depends on the tastes of each one. The idea is to enjoy the process.

Finger penetration.

When your partner is comfortable, you can begin finger penetration. Better said, with just one and always well lubricated. To penetrate, you do not have to put your finger like someone who is pressing their nose, it should be slowly and with the tip as if we wanted to capture the

fingerprint, thus avoiding scratching with the nails; it is preferable to do it with short nails if you have no experience.
It is important that the sphincter be releasing on its own, not forcing it.
So, we are dilating and relaxing it. If you do not relax, it's because we're going too fast.
Remember to always be attentive to the reactions of your partner's body.

Insert the penis or sex toy.

When finger penetration is pleasant for your partner, we can move on to inserting the penis or a toy (dildos, prostate massagers, plugs, anal beads), but remember that for rich anal sex, you do not need a very deep penetration. Simply inserting the tip of the limb or accessory is sufficient. Later you will gain the taste and confidence to deepen the penetration and explore other pleasures of anal sex.

What hygienic considerations should I consider when practicing anal sex?

To answer this question, I will make a list of the most common recommendations and those that I consider most important, but if you want more information about it, you can check more sources.
Clean the area, washing it with soap and water is enough. You can lightly insert a finger during cleaning to rinse the inside a little.
Emptying the intestine is a personal option, although it is true that generally the stool is in a deeper part of the body, it is possible that the stimulation leaves some uncomfortable remains.
To avoid them, enemas with lukewarm water with a shower or anal cleansing bulb.
Bacteria that are harmful to the delicate vaginal / urological flora live within the intestine.
The ideal way to avoid infection is the use of a condom.
Follow the classic order of penetration mouth-vagina-anus, mouth-anus, or vagina-anus, to avoid infections.
Remember that if there is an exchange of fluids there is a risk of contagion of sexually transmitted diseases. For the anus too. You must take care.

Most extravagant fetishes

Sex fetishes have been around since ancient times. And while they were a taboo subject for many decades, many are no longer so strange today. However, it all depends on the person or the couple.

They help to break the sexual routine and, in turn, can lead to the experimentation of new sensations and experiences or, to magnify them. Now what are fetishes? Well, in erotic arousal or facilitation and achievement of orgasm, using a garment or object by a specific part of the body.

Anyone can have a fetish, just like sexual fantasies. However, there are some that are extravagant and that, although they seem unreal, are part of the sexual lives of many people in the world.

1. Ursusagalamatophilia

The ursusagalamatophilia is a filia that consists of dressing like a stuffed animal Although it seems extravagant and weird, it has become an immensely popular and practiced fetish.

In countries like the United States there are groups in which the members are dressed in this way. Even in Japan, there is an anime (cartoon series) based on this filia.

2. Salirophilia

Most people worry about having a good hygiene routine before having sex; however, for others, hygiene or the smell of a perfume may not have anything erotic about it.

There are those who enjoy and are excited by the idea of getting dirty during sex, or else, dirtying their partner. This can range from ruffling the companion, to smearing makeup and ripping their clothes.

Usually, along with this fetish, fantasies of domination and submission are accompanied.

3. Infantilism paraphilic.

It refers to the fetish of wearing diapers and carrying out baby behaviors. Those who have it experience a great desire to be treated like little children.

The diaper gives them pleasure, security, and calm, whether it is introduced into sexual play.

It is more common in men than women.

4. Hematophilia

This filia corresponds to those who want to have a relationship similar to the romantic stories of vampires; Although it seems unreal, it is not far from the behaviors and fetishes of many couples. Its popularity even increased after the success of the Twilight saga and the vampire series derived from the film.

Hematophilia consists of involving, using, or even taking blood during sexual intercourse, or having any erotic thoughts with it.

Hemophilia (inherited disorder) should not be confused with hematophilia (fetish).

5. Claustrophilia

While some feel panicky in closed spaces (claustrophobia), others feel a high degree of sexual arousal when they are with their partners in tight and small spaces.

This fetish is more common than many think, and those who have it often take advantage of places, like the bathroom (or the shower, to be more specific), to satisfy their sexual desires.

6. Autoandrophilia

It is a bit of a weird fetish, but it is common. The woman takes pleasure in dressing as a man and acting as such during foreplay and intercourse.

Autoandrophilia can occur in both heterosexual and homosexual women.

7. Somnophilia

It is also known as the "Sleeping Beauty fetish" and is characterized by arousal and orgasm while the couple is asleep.

Some only need to see and caress to feel pleasure; others, on the other hand, go so far as to masturbate and even practice sexual intercourse while their partner sleeps. What is exciting is the euphoria that fear produces when discovered. However, it also has to do with having someone under control and totally subdued.

8. Agalmatophilia

The attraction to mannequins is known as agalmatophilia and refers to the excitement produced by the immobility of dolls or statues. Many people even steal or buy mannequins for the sole purpose of having sex with them.

9. Formicphilia

This is perhaps one of the most extravagant and rare fetishes out there. It consists of enjoying sexually having insects crawling on the body. The favorite areas of people who have this taste include the genitals and erogenous parts such as the breasts or the neck.

10 tips for masturbation as a couple

One of the most frequent complaints among couples is that their sexual interactions have become routine and unsatisfactory due, in general, to stress and daily obligations. When it comes to innovating and improving the quality of intimate exchanges, everything is valid. However, there is a resource that is as relevant as it is forgotten: masturbation as a couple.

There are still many myths and taboos around masturbation. Some even feel hurt, upset, or rejected if their partner resorts to solo masturbation. However, it is a totally healthy and natural practice that can benefit you in several ways.

Benefits of masturbation as a couple.
Masturbation as a couple is a way to bond. Increase trust and intimacy.

Masturbation as a couple allows you to discover the other and allow yourself to be discovered, even to connect on a deeper level. It is a practice in which you are usually more present, more aware of the sensations. And, although it can make certain people feel vulnerable, the degree of intimacy and trust that is achieved is much greater.

Promotes communication and knowledge of the other.

Many of the sexual difficulties of a couple are caused by a lack of assertive communication. Being able to convey to the other what you want and like is essential; as well as being willing to listen and learn. Masturbation as a couple offers you the perfect opportunity to observe, guide and be guided when it comes to giving and receiving pleasure.

Increase satisfaction.

At times, you may think that intercourse and penetration are essential and mandatory. It is common to believe that they are the target and that everything else does not matter. But it is necessary to generate a sufficient degree of desire and excitement for sexual intercourse to be satisfactory. And, for this, masturbation as a couple is an excellent tool.

Create a suitable environment.

Desire is nourished by stimulations of all kinds, and a conducive and suggestive environment can make the experience much more pleasant. Thus, find a comfortable, intimate, and quiet place, and spend some time preparing it. Lower the light, light some candles, play background music, or use aromatherapy are some options.

No rules

Remember that this moment is only for you and your partner and should be tailored to your preferences. You can take off your clothes or keep them on, caress each other or facing each other, use sex toys or not. There are no rules, you always choose.

Try and learn.
One of the biggest advantages of this practice is that it allows you to get to know your partner better and, also, make yourself known. Allow yourself to try and explore new sensations, keep an eye on the other's reactions and your own and you will mutually discover your tastes and preferences.

Communicate

Regarding the above, it is also essential that both of you can communicate assertively. The other is not able to read your mind, so you must convey your opinions and suggestions.

Likewise, you must know how to listen and let yourself be guided without feeling attacked or rejected.

Think less, feel more.

It is essential that during this period you can "disconnect your mind" and connect with your body. Fears, prejudices, and worries can ruin the moment and prevent you from enjoying yourself. So, focus on your breath, on the sensations that come and let yourself go.

Do not be in a hurry.

For masturbation as a couple to be pleasant it is important to approach it as an end. Do not try to seek and achieve orgasm at all costs, go easy and delight in the process.

Do not look for perfection.

If this is the first time you have tried this experience with your partner, it is likely that the result is far from perfect. But this is not necessary and should not discourage you. Over time, each other's knowledge and mutual trust will increase, and the results will be more positive.

Repeat and innovate!

Finally, try to introduce partner masturbation as a frequent element in your sex life. It is useless to try one day and leave forever. Make it part of the routine, innovate in environments, postures, or means of stimulation.

How to masturbate a woman correctly

The pursuit of pleasure is one of the main objectives of the human being, and sexual pleasure is no exception. In fact, sexual satisfaction is closely related to the well-being of the couple.

However, over the years, monotony, and a decrease in dedication to the sexual needs of the couple can cause their satisfaction to be affected.

Masturbation is a good alternative to increase sexual pleasure in intimate relationships and it has its advantages and benefits.

And since some men may wonder how to masturbate a woman properly, in this article we have put together a list of 19 steps to answer this question. They are as follows.

1. Locate the clitoris.

Despite having different sexual organs, both men and women can have really pleasant orgasms. Now, while the penis only has one way to transport sensations to the brain, the female genital tract has three or four. Without a doubt, the best known is the clitoris: a small, fleshy body that is found in the highest part of the vulva.

Stimulating the clitoris correctly can lead women to experience extremely pleasant sensations. Now, it is necessary to know how to do it, and not to stimulate directly if there is not enough excitement.

2. And the G-spot.

Much is said about the G-spot, and surely everyone knows that this is the magic button for women. The G-spot is still the internal part of the clitoris as research indicates, so it is an area that we must stimulate if we want to masturbate a woman correctly.

To locate it, it is necessary to insert the finger with the nail upside down and, once inside, lift the tip so that the finger is hooked. Then you will detect a protruding area inside, a kind of button.

3. Stimulate both at the same time.

To increase the pleasurable sensations, it is possible to play with two hands (or even just one) to stimulate both the external clitoris and the G-spot. Sensations to the limit if you can perform a combined movement.

4. Don't just focus on the clitoris.

Now, in the vagina there are other erogenous zones, so you can experience what sensations touching them produces. Surely the person with whom you are having intimate relationships can give you feedback on what they like.

5. Explore the body.

To produce a more pleasant stimulation, it is important to know that there are other erogenous zones that can be stimulated. For example, while stimulating the clitoris, the neck can be a great ally to increase sensations. Also stimulate the anal area. It is important to think of the body as a whole, as it is a great treasure in its entirety.

6. Use lubricant.

When masturbating a woman, it is ideal to use a lubricant, thus increasing pleasure and avoiding pain. 50 percent of a recent survey stated that lubrication helped them achieve orgasm,

7. Invest in a sex toy.

Masturbation not only includes fingers, but it is possible to do it with other objects, for example, with vibrators. There are many on the market, so you can do your research before choosing one.

8. Or maybe two.

One sex toy can be a good alternative, but two is even better. Do not be shy and use them at the same time. Orgasm can be even more pleasant.

9. Play with the environment

The place where you carry out masturbation can also be decisive in promoting a climate of trust and relaxation. Perhaps you can decorate the room with candles and induce relaxation with music that invites you to let yourself go.

10. Get to know the other person.

Take your time to get to know the other person, because not everyone has the same tastes.

11. Keep communicating.

So, you can ask him directly and keep communication fluent. In this way it is possible to improve things and achieve much more intense sensations.

12. Be gentle and gradually increase the intensity.

We may think that by giving more intensity we will achieve greater orgasms, but the truth is that increasing the intensity is the ideal. In fact, an especially useful technique is to delay the climax.

13. Vary touch and movement.

Make circular movements, in a straight line, rub, massage, blow, in other words, vary the movements and the touch on the clitoris and other erogenous zones. This can help create very pleasant sensations.

14. Don't forget your nipples.

The nipples, like the genitals, have many nerve endings that help increase female arousal. However, many men do not know how to take advantage of it, as they are too rough. In this erogenous zone, it is important to be delicate.

15. Use your imagination and get lost in the present

These tips can be very useful, but the key is to lose yourself in the moment, connect with the other person and understand the situation at that moment. So, pay attention to what is happening between you and focus on what you are doing.

16. Try other places.

Although before I have commented that it is necessary to create a favorable climate for intimate relationships, it is not only necessary to think about the room. It is possible to be creative or to look for other places that can stimulate the senses, for example, in the bathtub.

17. Try different games.

It is also possible to try different games or postures, or to add stimuli to sexual play, for example by adding ice, as the cold can intensify the sensations.

18. Try different postures.

Masturbation can also be carried out from different positions. Therefore, you do not have to be closed-minded, and you can attack from different angles.

19. Don't stop, go on ...

Women can have multiple orgasms, meaning they can have a sequence of orgasms one after the other without going through the resolution stage. Therefore, even if you think that you are in the climax, do not stop and continue ...

How to masturbate a man.

There are many theories about what men like in bed, but one thing is clear, and that is that masturbation is always one of the most effective and enjoyable techniques. If you have ever wondered how to masturbate a man so that he enjoys like never before, we make it easy for you.

If a few years ago sex was basically limited to missionary and kissing, today there are countless ways to enjoy and make your boy enjoy. One of them is male masturbation, a practice older than fire (probably) but one that women find it hard to get the hang of for, basically, anatomical reasons.

Written may seem theoretical and unsightly, but in practice success is assured.

1. The proper posture.

Correct posture will make the difference between clumsy work and an experience that takes you to the height of ecstasy. You can try different positions and then ask him which one he liked the most. The first thing you should make sure is if he likes to stand or sit better. That is something for him to decide or leave it up to the situation in which you find yourself.

Next, you must be clear about where you are. Do not be afraid, try different variants first. Do not be shy about changing positions to find which one works best, her breathing and her face will give you the best clue. The best thing about masturbation is precisely that feeling of control you have over him: you will be the active part. You decide what will happen and how it will happen, and you will love that!

Another thing you can do is grab him from behind. Thus, you will let your imagination and fantasy fly and, as you decide how far to go, you will have it delivered to you. Also, if you squeeze it hard during the act, you will create a more intimate and sensual experience. Be careful, of course, with squeezing too much or squeezing the testicles, you should only do that if he asks you to.

2. Key factor to masturbate a man: spontaneity.

The best thing about masturbation is that it is easy to carry out anytime, anywhere. For this reason, it makes it the perfect technique in situations where a quick response is necessary. That is, in those in which you want to pamper your partner giving him instant pleasure. You can do it anywhere: at home, in the elevator, in a parking lot ... But if you give free rein to passion, make sure no one sees you!

You can also hold him lovingly in the shower. Get into it, hold it from behind and, with a little lather in your hands, gently massage it.

Spontaneity is a very sexy thing, so do not be afraid to surprise your partner whenever you want. To find out if you feel like it at that moment, start with a game. Lightly caress her thighs. Little by little, he unzips his pants. If he does not do anything to stop you, it means he is wanting it. Another place to try is in the car ... Try these poses and discover how comfortable and sexy they can be.

3. Use your whole hand.

You are already in position. Now is the time to figure out how to grip his penis. It is
not totally necessary to use all five fingers since having a free pair of fingers allows
certain games to be played: use three fingers for the upper part, and the lower two for
the testicles. In this way, your partner will feel more in contact with you. Don't forget,
the best manual pleasure, like sex in general, doesn't just center around the penis.

Most men like to feel pressure during masturbation but remember that you are holding
one of the most sensitive parts of your body, so do not overdo it. If you are not
entirely sure how much pressure to apply, use different grasping techniques and watch
the reaction. Or, even easier, ask him if he wants you to make it stronger or softer.

4. Constant rhythm

It's time to grab it and get started. Move your hand in a steady motion until you notice
how you like it. Start off with a slow, smooth movement and see changing the pace to
make it a little faster, but not too much, unless you see that he likes it. Many men
prefer a stronger movement the further away from the body the hand is, and softer
when it approaches the root of the penis. However, it can cause pain if the skin is
stretched too much. So, watch out for the jerks!

The best way to find the right rhythm is to let your partner put his hand on yours and
guide you through the movement he prefers, at least the first time. It is important not
to lose rhythm or strength, once you start, because it is this movement performed
repeatedly that will make you climax.

5. Use both hands!

If you want to be a manual art professional, you must exploit your multitasking
capabilities. It may seem difficult, but you will achieve it in no time. Put one hand on
his member and with the other pay attention to his nipples or his testicles: caressing
and massaging them can lead your partner to a very intense orgasm. They are highly
erogenous zones, although make sure he likes you to touch both zones, since there is
nothing written about tastes.

6. Especially soft

Anything that reduces the friction between your hands and his penis should be
considered. Using oil or lubricant will reduce any discomfort your boy may feel. You
will increase the desire and desire to play. If you choose to lubricate your penis with

gel or oil, you will achieve that your movements are more intense and pleasant, greater sensitivity and less effort with better results. With some of these products you can even rub his glans, perhaps the most sensitive (and potentially pleasant) area of the male body. Test it!

7. Games and toys

Sex toys, or certain everyday accessories will help you a lot to stimulate different areas. Try a vibrating ring or simply play with the textures: caress the penis with a velvet glove or with your hand smeared in some oil. In addition, there are various sex toys for men and, more specifically, for penises, which allow to lengthen the erection or stimulate it in different ways. If you add these toys to some of the hottest erotic games, fun and diversity is guaranteed.

8. Discover your erogenous zones.

No two men are the same or two men who like exactly the same. However, if we generalize, there are a couple of pleasure areas common to all that you should know. One is the tip of the penis, as we have just mentioned, and another is the perineum, that is, the area between the penis and the anus. With a little pressure, you can stimulate your G-spot, the prostate, in this way. In this way, making her reach an intense orgasm is a matter of time. And, by the way, try English too, many love it.

9. Stronger?

Novels like Fifty Shades of Gray have focused on an increasingly common fantasy: rough sex. If you and your boy want to try, do not hesitate to find out a little better about these practices and start from less to more, as in the positions in the gallery that we show you below. If your boy likes this type of practice, he will love that you masturbate him harder than conventional, so try squeezing harder, tucking your fingers on the testicles, or nibbling on his neck and nipples while you masturbate him.

Love moorings- Easy and Powerful.

Sometimes it is difficult to get a woman's attention through normal contact. I understand you perfectly because this has already happened to me. So, in this article I want to share with you some highly effective and simple spells to fall in love with a woman that worked for me, and that I am sure will be particularly useful for you.

Everything is fair in love, right? So, it is totally valid to use spells to make a woman fall in love. In this way, you will resort to powerful forces, that you cannot even imagine, so that that girl who drives you crazy falls at your feet.

For some spells you will need some materials, and for others you can practically execute without materials.

Some of the spells will help you to get love from her indefinitely, while others will get you to attract her temporarily. Let's see:

1. White magic to seduce and dominate a difficult woman.

"I want you to notice me" is the typical request I receive in the mail. And I want you to stay calm because, with this simple white witchcraft procedure, you are going to achieve it even if initially I have not paid much attention to you.

I want you to fully trust the process that I am going to reveal to you and execute it to the letter. They are enormously powerful, so be incredibly careful about your wishes:

Necessary materials:

A photo of her.

A small stamp of San Antonio.

A pencil with erasures.

A deep plate.

Sugar.

Sea salt.

Sunflower oil.

White candle.

Process:

Write her full name behind the Saint Anthony stamp.

Take the photo of your girl and paste it on the same side where you wrote her name.

Pass the pencil eraser over the photo so that it is completely sealed with the stamp.

Spread the sugar in the bowl and add the sea salt.

Add about 3 drops of sunflower oil.

Place the photo in the middle, and next to it, place the white candle. You can put it on a plate or a base to avoid accidents.

Light the candle every night, and extinguish it the next morning, until it is completely consumed.

After lighting it each night, say the following prayer:

San Antonio de Padua, help me to get the love of [pronounces his name and surname], since I want him to be my sentimental partner. I promise to protect and love her so that she may be happy for the rest of our lives.

2. How to bewitch a woman using semen.

The energy that has an orgasm is extraordinarily strong. For that reason, we are going to use sperm to increase your level of attraction:

Necessary materials:

Your semen.

Your saliva.

A ceramic vase.

Process:

As you orgasm to get your sperm, focus on your goal. Visualize your beloved and imagine the 2 together.

Pour your semen into the ceramic glass.

Add your saliva.

Pronounce the following words:

My passion will ignite the love in you: [pronounces her name], I will make you think of me, and love me day and night. My sperm will inevitably attract you. So be it.

In this way you will be able to modify his sensation, and he will have the need to get closer to you. You will notice a special behavior in her in the next 5 days.

3. Witchcraft to make a woman fall in love with her underwear.

This time you are going to use black magic. It is a bit more complicated than the previous 2 options since you will need your underwear and hers. Let's see everything you will need:

Necessary materials:

Your underwear

Underwear of your beloved.

Red thread and needle.

Two red candles.

A white candle.

A medium container.

Mineral water.

Process:

Call your girl under any pretext, the goal is for her to keep thinking of you. Do not force the conversation to inevitably think of you either. You can talk about anything; her subconscious will be left with the last action that will have been talking to you.

Do not allow more than 2 hours to start the ritual.

On a table, place the 3 candles so that they form a triangle. You can place them in any order. The important thing is the triangle.

Light the candles.

In the middle of the triangle, place the container, fill it halfway with mineral water.

Take the intimate garments of both and start sewing them with the thread and the needle so that both garments are together.

When you finish joining the two garments, submerge them in the water.

For 15 minutes, stare at the water while visualizing the two of you together. Imagine both of you as you wish a normal day would be between the two of you.

Attention! first remove the container from the triangle, and then extinguish the candles.

Remove the garments from the container and store them somewhere where only you have access. no one should see them.

The tied garments should ALWAYS keep them.

4. How to cast a spell on an older or married woman.

Women usually like to be with an older man, so if you want to break that stigma, I recommend that you use the following spell:

Necessary materials:

A tablespoon of cinnamon.

A photo of the woman you want to attract.

A tablespoon of honey

A stick of incense.

A folio, or a blank sheet, of A4 size (that is, a plain white paper).

A few drops of your usual perfume.

An envelope.

A red pen.

Some matches or matches.

A large container.

Process:

Light the incense.

Draw a big heart on the paper, using the red pen.

Inside the heart write the first name and first surname of your loved one.

On the edge of the heart, smear the honey.

Spread the cinnamon in the same contour of the honey.

Add a few drops of your perfume on the name of your future wife.

Kiss the photo of her and envision a future moment together.

Put the photo aside. Fold the paper and put it in the envelope.

Finally add the photo. Be careful, it must be in that order: first the paper and then the photo.

Place the envelope on the container and burn it with the matches (or matches).

While the envelope is burning, repeat the following 3 times:

We will always be united by this heat, and we will become inseparable.

In less than 1 week you will notice a growing interest from her for you.

5. Spell of the box

You have here a simple and agile formula for you to feed your existence with that conquest that you crave for your life. It is an amazingly effective love tie if you follow the following steps to the letter:

Necessary materials:

An updated photo of you

A photo of the boy (if you do not have a photo or know his name, he writes on a paper some reference that represents him, as well as the boy from the store)

Red thread, representing destiny.

Scissors

Box or container where to place the two photos.

Brown sugar

Process:

Take both photos (or whatever you have prepared).

Top one on top of the other and trim the excess so that both are even and the same size.

Place the images inward and then you will see them around with the red destiny thread.

In the box or container, place the brown sugar up to the middle of the pot.

Locate the stitched photos on the sugar.

So, recite the following words, with great faith:

May this spell so that he thinks of me, I become the protagonist of your most adorable thoughts, until our love is consumed.

You will complete, filling the container with the rest of the sugar on the photos, until they are completely covered, closing the pot, and putting it in a secret and safe place.

When the spell has taken effect, you must try to get the recipient of your heart to consume the sugar you used in the coffee or other infusion. That is transcendental so that the person in question falls into your arms for life.

6. Ishtar's Spell

This is a ritual for me to call you, too powerful that you must fervently believe in. It is exclusively for women and must take place on a Tuesday or Saturday at midnight. To put it into practice:

Necessary materials:

1 photo of the person

1 white or red bag

Incense

2 red candles

Honey

Process:

You must light the incense at least 1 hour before performing the spell.

Light the candles carefully.

Take the photo and pass it through the fire without burning it or touching it.

Spread the face of the person photographed with some honey and place the two burning candles on the photo.

Concentrated and with great devotion you will say these words converted into prayer:

In the mighty name of Ishtar, who has accompanied human beings since ancient times. You who with your strength decide who triumphs and who is defeated, praised Ishtar, listen to my plea, I am unhappy, and I turn to you. Make (mention recipient's name) think of me day and night. I want to be her greatest wish, goddess of love, please, so be it.

Blow out the candles and put the photo inside the bag that you will keep there for a month until your wish is positively fulfilled.

7. Using vinegar

A ritual for me to call you and desperately look for you is this that I am capturing here for you. Do it outdoors, in the morning or at night, never in the afternoon. Adaptable to men and women, here it goes:

Necessary materials:

5 white candles

1 photo of the person

Sherry vinegar

Coarse salt

Process:

Draw a circle on the ground with the salt, in such a way that both of your legs enter.

Arrange the 5 lit candles around the circle.

Place the photo inside the circle and put vinegar on the body and face on the image.

You stand inside the circle drawn with the salt, raise your hands and speak like this:

Kerobal, I call you to help me with your power, inhabitant of darkness. Hear my plea, make (mention the name of the one offering your wish) feel totally attracted to me. Kerobal, you have here this humble mortal who believes in you. So be it.

Blow out the candles and bury the photograph.

When the wish is granted, where you buried that photo, do the same with a dried fruit as a sign of gratitude.

There are many more spells for him to call you today or to write to you asking for the attention you are looking for to share with him. You must learn to perform these magic procedures, with the faith and concentration necessary to succeed in your wishes.

Do not stop believing in yourself when you do it, because you are worth a lot, if he deserves you, he will come into your life very soon to start an idyll of two, full of romantic experiences. And happiness will be with you!

8. Spell to make a man fall in love.
This ritual will help you fall in love with the man you want, the man you have wanted to have for so long but for some reason does not resolve to be with you. Just do it with great faith and remember the main ingredient of all spells. "Faith"

Materials:

1. A beer

2. An apple

3. Four pins

4. A photograph of the man you want to fall in love with

5. A plastic bowl

6. A knife

7. A piece of red cloth

8. Three white candles

In order to start with this spell, it is especially important that you know that you must know the man you want to fall in love with, it cannot be a man you meet on social networks and you have not had physical contact with him, that is, it must be someone with whom you share a lot of time to that can work as you want.

If you are thinking of doing it to make Kim Kardashian or Brad Pitt fall in love, I regret to inform you that it will not work for you, do you agree?

You are going to add all the beer in the plastic container, then put the whole apple in the beer for an hour.

After that hour you are going to remove the red apple and you are going to split it in half and with the knife you are going to put the photograph of the man you want to fall in love within the middle of the apple and then with the four pins you are going to join the two halves of the Apple.

Once the apple is joined with the photograph in the middle, you are going to wrap the apple in the piece of red cloth and proceed to bury it next to a leafy tree, full of life.

And for three nights you are going to visit the place where you buried the apple, and you are going to kneel in the place, and you are going to say with your eyes closed the following words with great faith.

You will fall in love with me (your full name) madly, you will think about my day and night, you will want my body like drinking water, may the energy of this tree fill my ritual with energy and allow me to fall in love with (Full name of the man you want fall in love), that he cannot live without me.

After those three nights going to the place where you buried the apple, you will see how that man you want so much begins to change his attitude with you, and the love for you begins to show, his desire to have you, when this man is completely with you, you will light three white candles and in your mind you will thank the spirits of love for having given you the opportunity to have that man you wanted so much by your side.

9. Spell to make a friend fall in love.

This ritual will make it easier for you to perform since being a friend of the person you want to fall in love with will make it easier for you to conquer them.
Through this spell to fall in love you can get closer to her and show her that you love her with her heart,
Besides being her friend, you will become her partner, when she has fallen in love with you there will be no going back.
This spell must be done on a Monday at any time, and it must be specifically that day since it is the eating of the week, the same as the eating of a special love between you and your friend or friend.
These are the materials you should use:
1. Two red candles.
2. White ribbon.
3. two white candles.
4. Red ribbon.
5. A blue ink marker.

To begin you are going to take the blue ink marker and on the red ribbon you are going to write your full name.
With the same blue ink marker, you are going to write on the white ribbon the full name of your friend, the girl you want to fall in love with you.
Then you are going to take the red ribbon on which you wrote your full name and you are going to join the two white candles with it.
You are going to do the same with the white ribbon on which you wrote your friend's name and you are going to join two red candles.
After having the candles together, you will proceed to light them and repeat the following words twice out loud.
I join you as I join these candles, I join you as I feel united to you, you fall in love with me as I do with you, we will have a relationship full of happiness and passion.

When the candles have been completely consumed, you will pick up what is left of the candles and the ribbons and you will put it under your mattress and little by little you will see how this woman stops being your friend and becomes your beloved and you in his beloved. When you sleep with her for the first time in your bed, the next day you're going to get everything out of her under her mattress and you're going to bury it and that's it! Now your friend is your girl.

spells to fall in love easy and fast:

10. Spell with white rose:
Take a white rose and strip it off. Put it on a red cloth while we say: "Through this action I attract you to my heart", think about the person we want to fall in love with. Put the red cloth with the rose petals in the right pocket. Wear it for three days.

11. Spell with candle and photo:
Take a photo of the person we want to fall in love with and put it on a table, light a red candle in front of the photo. Say: "By means of this spell, I spell this love." Stay silent for five minutes. Blow out the candle. Do the spell again until the candle goes out on different days, all in a row. Don't cut the spell.

12. Spell to fall in love with pink paper:
Take a pink paper, write the name of the person we want to fall in love with. While we do it say the name of that person three times. Then put the paper in our purse or wallet and take it there for a week. At the end of the week, take the paper and put it under our pillow, use it under the pillow for a week, then take the paper and burn it, by making it say: "I book you everything, you are mine."

13. Spell to fall in love with glass of water and lemon:
Take a glass and fill it with pure water if it is mineral water better. Put the glass on a table, and then put three drops of lemon in the water. By making him say: "From now on you are mine." Then leave the glass for three days in the open. After those three days, take a tablespoon of that water and put it in another glass of water, add mineral water until the glass is full and repeat the procedure. Leave three days and then throw the water into a stream or a

lake, that is to say, to any natural water source. If you do not have it nearby you can throw the
water into the pool and run the water.

14.Full moon spell to fall in love:
This spell must be done with a full moon. Being out in the open looking at the moon, it does
not matter if it is cloudy, but you must be able to locate it in the sky and look at it. Think of
the person you want to fall in love with, raise your arms and breathe deeply, say: "Moon,
mother, sister, by feminine power I summon the forces of light so that he can come closer."
Lower your arms and breathe deeply thinking about him. Do not stay much longer low the
moon.

15. Spell with three red candles to fall in love:
Take three red candles and form a triangle. Put a paper in the center that has the name of the
person you want to fall in love with. Light the candles. Think about what we want to attract
that person. Remain silent until the candles are gone. Store the paper in your underwear
drawer.

16. Spell with two photos to fall in love:
Take two photos, one of you and the other of the person you want to fall in love with, put
them on a table, draw a heart with a red pen so that it occupies the two photos, when doing
so, say the following words: "I will join you forever.". Keep the two photos in your wallet or
in a pocket, by doing so stick the photos with an adhesive tape.

17. Spell with photo and underwear:
Take your underwear and fold it as best you can. Then take a photo of the person you want to
fall in love with and tie it with a thread to your underwear. By doing so say. "You are mine
now." Carry that little package everywhere in your purse or in a pocket. No one should see it.
Highly effective in awakening passion.

18. Spell with sugar and cinnamon to fall in love:
Take a little cinnamon stick and put it on the fire so that it lights a little. Throw sugar over the
cinnamon until the heat is extinguished. As you do so, say the following words: "You come
closer to me, you are mine, and I yours." Put that cinnamon that will be sugary in a glass of

water. Leave the glass of water overnight by your bed. Think about it before sleeping. Throw the water with the cinnamon in a place that nobody can find it, if it is necessary to bury it.

19. Spell with hair:

Get a hair or a group of them, from the person you want to fall in love with. Put the hair in a glass that has a little alcohol so that the hair is submerged in it. When putting the hair say: "You dissolve in my desire and you are mine." Take the glass and move it a little, repeating this phrase three times. Leave the glass overnight in the light of the moon, then the next day remove the hair and burn it, repeating the same phrase. Throw the alcohol on the ground.

20. SPELL WITH SUGAR TO FALL IN LOVE WITH A MAN

Conquer that man's heart with this simple spell. Learn this ritual to tie a man! With this spell to make a man fall in love with sugar, you will make that man's heart open and be much more receptive to the messages you send him. His attitude will be much more loving and pleasant. You will have paved the way to enter his heart!

What materials will you need to perform the sugar love spell to conquer a man?
Sugar.
A red candle.
An incense candle.
A white paper.
A grain of pepper.
How to perform a love spell with sugar to conquer a man

1. We will begin by taking the sheet of paper, on which we will write the name of the man we want to conquer; below we will put ours and we will enclose them within a red circle.
2. On the back of the paper we will write: "Love me as I love you, our love will unite us forever." You will turn the paper over again with the names facing up and you will add a little sugar inside the red circle along with the peppercorn.
3. Once the previous step is done, we will fold the paper only once and place the red candle on top.
4. We will light the candle and let it burn until the first drop of wax falls on the folded paper. Then we will extinguish the candle, we will fold the paper again, taking care that neither the sugar nor the peppercorn falls off and we will put it in a bag.

5. We will have that bag for three nights under the pillow we sleep on. On the fourth night we will light an incense candle and let the paper burn completely.

6.When it is consumed, we will take the ashes and carefully scatter them to the wind whispering the following phrase repeatedly: «Love me as I love you, our love will unite us forever. With this love spell we will get the man who receives it to begin to have feelings of affection and interest towards us. He will awaken the most sensitive side of him and break his armor, with what our emotions will end up moving to his heart. His sexual desire will also be activated on the person doing the ritual, beginning to feel attracted not only emotionally but also physically.

21 LOVE SPELL WITH LEMON AND SUGAR

Are you attracted to a man who has not yet noticed you? Quiet. With this love spell with lemon and sugar you will be able to capture all his attention.

Take note of the necessary materials:

A lemon.
Rose petals.
Red ribbon.
Red candle.
Sugar.
Process:

First, we will cut the lemon into two parts. While performing this action recite the following text aloud: «I cut your indifference. I tie you with the red ribbon of love and passion. "
Put the halved lemon on a plate and pour honey while you pronounce: "I attract you like flowers to the bee, you see me sweet and attractive."
Then he sprinkles sugar and repeats the following sentence three times in a row: "Only love, affection and sweetness do you want to give me."
Then he circles the rose petals around the plate.
Finally, he lights the red candle with wooden matches and watches the flame for fifteen minutes while you think about that man.

These two spells with sugar to conquer a man are ideal, but there are many other homemade spells to fall in love that you can learn to find the one that best suits your situation. In addition, you can always consult the tarot if you need answers about the feelings of your loved one.

How to increase libido.

Problems associated with decreased sexual desire should be addressed by professionals in the field. However, there are some natural remedies that help counteract them.
Is it possible to increase libido naturally? How is it done? What benefits could it bring? These are some questions that people who currently experience low libido ask themselves.

Lack of libido or sexual loss of appetite can have different causes: emotional issues, stress, nutritional deficiencies, psychological disorders, side effects of medications, hormonal irregularities, among others.
Faced with this problem, it is important to consult your family doctor, a psychosexual therapist, a contraception and sexual health clinic and other entities that can provide everything you need to overcome it.

First, it must be considered that the lack of sexual desire can have various causes and, therefore, they must be recognized and given appropriate treatment according to the case.
As a complement, you can try some remedies of natural origin whose properties help increase libido. Which are? How do you make it? Here we detail it.
The prototype of the woman who, after a certain age, suffers a decrease in libido is today an anecdote. Modern life, characterized by a stressful routine and a poor diet, can cause libido problems, among many other health problems.

For this reason, it is important to do self-criticism, analyze the possible causes of sexual loss of appetite and put a solution to it at the hands of professionals. In this way we will improve our state of health in general, while we manage to have an active and healthy sexual life.

Cinnamon with honey

Cinnamon is a spice with a delicious and aromatic flavor with stimulating and calorific properties, two virtues highly appreciated by those who suffer from a lack of libido. In addition, if we combine it with honey, rich in vitamins and minerals, we get a very nutritious remedy that gives us a large dose of energy and vitality.

Every morning we will take a tablespoon of honey with Ceylon cinnamon powder. We have chosen this variety because it is the one that contains the most medicinal properties, even though its price is a little more expensive than the rest.

Nowadays, fruit and vegetable smoothies are in fashion, since they allow us to consume raw and nutritious food, with all its properties, in a comfortable and pleasant way. These shakes are rich in vitamins, minerals, fiber, protein, and fatty acids, making them ideal to increase the feeling of energy.

In this case, we suggest adding a little powdered maca, an ingredient that has become popular for its aphrodisiac properties.

Although the evidence in this regard is limited and contradictory

point out that its consumption has been promoted to improve sexual desire and sperm count, mood, as well as energy and physical endurance.

Note: those who suffer from high blood pressure or nervousness should consult a doctor before consuming maca.

Ylang-ylang essential oil

Essential oils are a natural and highly effective resource to enhance the sensuality in the couple and increase the libido in a natural way. These oils can be used as perfumes, to aromatize the bedroom or to perform massages.

Ylang-ylang essential oil is one of the most aphrodisiac, along with vanilla, jasmine, cinnamon or ginger.

This oil can be used in aromatherapy to reduce anxiety, depression, and high blood pressure.

All this, in general, is beneficial when it comes to increasing sexual desire. Remember that, many times, the lack of libido comes from an uncontrolled mood.

Ginger in all recipes

Ginger supplementation, particularly under conditions of oxidative stress, is suggested to improve testosterone production in men. However, the evidence is still limited. We can add ginger to all kinds of recipes: Bread. Lemonade. Juices and smoothies. Sweets and cakes. Meat and fish.

Laminaria

Laminar is a type of algae rich in B vitamins, minerals, fiber, and protein. It includes different varieties, such as kombu or fucus, all of them greatly beneficial to remineralize the body and improve health. One of the most unknown virtues of these algae is to increase sexual desire.

Bach flowers

The evidence on the efficacy of Bach flowers is limited and controversial. In fact, there is no research that associates its use with an increase in sexual desire.

However, in popular culture they have been used as an aphrodisiac, especially in aromatherapy. In this way, it also helps to reduce emotional imbalances.

Chocolate, a delight to increase libido naturally.

Chocolate is one of the foods that is associated with increased sexual desire. Since ancient times it has been used to increase energy level and libido.

This ingredient promotes the release of phenylethylamine and serotonin in the body.

Because of this, it is often considered an aphrodisiac and energetic. In general, it lifts the mood and reduces states of stress and depression.

Is it possible to turn to the remedies and the sexologist?

Yes, in the face of any problem associated with a decrease in sexual desire, it is best to consult with professionals in the field. Thus, it is more likely to determine its exact origin and the safest and most effective solution.

It should not be forgotten that, in addition to the doctor, the sexologist can provide useful instructions for day-to-day life.

As a complement to a healthy lifestyle, you can use the natural remedies that we have discussed above, however, although we can support ourselves with several natural remedies when wanting to increase libido, we must always maintain the corresponding precautions.

Tricks to increase your sexual desire today.

We live in a time of great demands and pressure and many times the first thing that suffers are our moments of enjoyment and enjoyment. Perhaps for different reasons, you have noticed that you are no longer the same as before and that your intimacy does not have the quality you want. Learn the secrets that can stimulate and improve your sex life.

What is libido?

It is the sexual desire of a person. There are also definitions such as that of the creator of psychoanalysis, the Austrian psychiatrist Sigmund Freud, who refers to libido as the psychic energy of a sexual nature that pushes for immediate satisfaction.

Desire psychology.

There are several reasons why you may feel the lack of sexual desire: work pressures, financial problems, routine in the couple and the passage of time are the most mentioned. Couples who manage to break with the routine are happier and longer lasting, but this requires work.

Logical fears.

Many fear that the vibrator could take away interest in the partner or sensitivity to the genital area. "While it is true that the intensity of the vibrator stimulation is unmatched, remember that it is not a replacement for your partner but an alternative to improve sexual enjoyment," explains Rampolla.

Texting.

The "hot" messages can go a long way in creating excitement and increasing passion. Shawn Edgington, author of "Reading Between the Lines: A Fun Guide to Simple and Stylish Texting" suggests that using bold text messages can keep the couple on fire.

Desire dresses in fashion.

Fashion aims to highlight lace and transparency. Black, white, and red are colors that are always in force, but also in the new trends are bright colors such as violet and animal print. There is also edible underwear, they are different tastes and smells.

Time to share.

Not everything is sex in the life of a couple. A report from the US National Library of Medicine argues that it is best for the couple to reserve some time for non-sexual intimacy, where they have time to talk or go out alone. This, in the long run, revives the sexual desire and interest in the other.

Communication and desire

Talking to your partner about what is going on is a good start to improving desire, experts from the Boston University Department of Sexual Medicine recommend. For them, caresses and words are important, for them a nice image and a sexy attitude are worth a thousand words.

Foods to Produce More Sperm

There are a lot of steps you can take to improve your sperm volume, and diet is undoubtedly one of the most important things that can help you increase your sperm count, as well as your semen volume. Here is a list of some foods that can help with this task.

Dark chocolate

 It is a powerful aphrodisiac, it contains L-Arginine. This is an amino acid that is known to increase semen volume, as well as enhance the intensity of orgasms.
Of course, do not overdo it or else the result will be weight gain that will only reduce the levels of testosterone in your body and your sperm count.

Oysters

Zinc is an essential mineral that plays an important role in improving testosterone levels as well as sperm production. Oysters are rich sources of this mineral.

An increase in testosterone levels also helps improve sexual desire and energy, which means that you will get more pleasure from your sexual encounters, as well as having a greater chance of conceiving.

Eggs
High in protein and vitamin E, eggs are considered to aid in the production of healthy and strong sperm in the testicles. It is also believed to protect sperm cells from the harmful effects of free radicals, which can eliminate sperm.

spinach
Another food to increase sperm is spinach. Green leafy vegetables like spinach are rich sources of folic acid. When folate levels are low, it can lead to malformed sperm being produced. This results in the sperm having difficulty reaching the egg and penetrating its protective barrier. Even if these sperm can fertilize an egg, the chances of birth defects are quite high in such cases.

Asparagus
Asparagus is a green vegetable rich in vitamin C. It is also a good food to increase sperm volume. Vitamin C protects sperm cells from the damaging effects of free radicals and thus ensures that sperm storage in the male reproductive system is not depleted.

Garlic
Garlic is an effective food that has been used for centuries to treat various physical ailments, such as heart problems and respiratory infections.
What many do not know is that it is also a powerful aphrodisiac and highly effective in boosting sperm volume.
It contains a compound called allicin that improves blood flow to male sex organs, increasing sperm production and semen volume.

Carrots
Vitamin A is an important nutrient for increasing sperm production, as well as improving its motility. Carrots are rich in this nutrient. You can also get vitamin A by eating foods like oatmeal, red bell peppers, and dried apricots.

These berries are known to improve general stamina and mood. But that is not all, it also keeps the temperatures in the scrotum at an optimal level.

The scrotum contains the testes that produce sperm.

Higher temperatures tend to hinder sperm production and decrease the volume that is released in a man's ejaculation. They also promote sperm production by improving blood circulation and protecting against free radical damage.

Walnuts

Another key nutrient for sperm volume is omega-3 fatty acids. These essential fatty acids are supposed to help increase sperm count, as well as improve blood flow in the penis. Including walnuts in your daily intake will help you produce more sperm.

Ginseng

Ginseng is a powerful herb known for its powerful effects on enhancing virility in men. It increases sexual desire and improves sexual performance.

It has been found to be very effective in men with erectile dysfunction, increased semen volume and sperm production.

This list of foods is certainly not too long. Eating a balanced diet (or taking a supplement for this purpose), which is rich in minerals such as zinc and vitamins such as A, B12, C, and folic acid, will ensure that a greater number of sperm are produced in the testicles. and are healthy enough to fertilize an egg.

Lifestyle changes that help produce more semen.

Daily exercise - Weight training is a great way to increase the secretion of testosterone in the body. Not only this, exercise also helps boost the flow of oxygenated blood that is rich in nutrients to the entire body, including the testicles. This will help your testicles get all the minerals necessary to increase sperm production.

Watch your diet - Obesity and unbalanced diets are some of the causes of health problems, including infertility (such as a low sperm count in men). Eating a balanced diet plays an important role in maintaining a healthy weight, this is an important part of an overall healthy life.

Quit Smoking

I know you already know that smoking causes cancer. However, what most men do not realize is that smoking is just as bad for sexual and reproductive health as well. Nicotine and other toxins in cigarettes can decrease sperm count and semen volume and also alter the DNA structure of sperm resulting in fertility problems. Therefore, you should consider quitting smoking.

Manage stress!

Stress, depression, and other negative feelings can wreak havoc on your body. Stress can release cortisol hormones into the bloodstream, which adversely impacts testosterone production. This negatively affects the production of semen. You should try to manage stress through yoga and other techniques like tai-chi, etc. Exercise is another effective stress buster.

Sex in the car: the 6 best positions to do it in the car.

When it comes to sex, there are many things we can explore, be it new poses, toys, oils, or tease games. But something that can always change the tone of our sex is the scenarios in which we practice it, so why not have sex in the car?

And the truth is that we do not know where that rush of excitement is going to catch us that we cannot resist. Why waste it just because we are not at home and we are in the car? Having sex in the car can be quite an adventure full of adrenaline and we will tell you the best positions to do it.

First tips to avoid dying trying.

Having sex in the car can be quite an adventure full of passion and adrenaline or a fiasco and a total disappointment if the proper precautions are not taken.

With this we are not telling you that you should carry a manual with you or that you should prepare it in advance, because that takes away all the emotion of spontaneity. But if you are presented with the opportunity to have sex in the car, there are certain precautions that you must consider at the moment.

Is it allowed in your country?

In many countries, having sex in the car is considered to be having sex in public space and is prohibited, so if you do not want to be embarrassed by the police in the middle of your moment of passion, make sure that they are not in full view and park the car in a more private place where they will not have problems.

Also make sure you have the doors closed properly, because even if they are in a very safe area, you do not want intrusions or unpleasant surprises in this moment of amazing privacy.

A little ventilation

Another tip that we give you before talking about the best positions for having sex in the car is to try to leave the windows open a little, thus preventing the windows from fogging up and allowing air circulation. Although you may not notice it because you are focused on your privacy, the air becomes concentrated and telltale scents can remain inside the car.

Also, when they finish having sex in the car, make sure there are no surprises out there and ventilate the car well, especially if it is your parents' car and not your own.

There are several positions for having sex in the car that you can experiment with, it all depends on the time you have, where you are, flexibility and desire. Choose your favorites!

1. Let's start with masturbation.

Although masturbation is not a position, it is the simplest way by which we can demonstrate our intentions to have sex in the car, since the way they are seated allows it very easily.

To masturbate your partner, just put your hand on his penis and start stroking him and very subtly open his pants and let him out, from then on you will surely know. Now, to allow your partner to touch you and masturbate you, you need to move forward a little so that your vagina does not get locked between your legs by your sitting position but is a little easier to access.

2. Now for oral sex

Another way to start sex in the car and get much more into action we could say is oral sex. If they are in the front seats it will be easier for you to simply lean over to where your partner is and perform oral sex.

Now in order for him to perform oral sex on you, they have to switch to the back seat. Once there, lie down mainly on the seat and spread your legs a little so that he, leaning on the seat on his knees, can perform oral sex on you.

3. The best posture: sitting facing him.

The best position to have sex in the car par excellence is that you sit on it looking at it from the front, especially if they do not have much time it is very easy to achieve this position and it will give them a lot of pleasure. When they are at it, try to recline the back of the chair to the maximum of it so that they can lie down, with you on it.

4. The classic missionary

The most traditional position in bed and that is never lacking can also be used to have sex in the car. Of course, it will have minimal variations that can be changed to become other positions.

If they are in the front of the car, they should fully recline the back of the passenger seat, so your guy can lie on top of you. It is not the most comfortable, especially if your boy is tall, but it is achieved.

Now, if they are in the back seat, it will be easier for you to lie on the chair and your boy to get on you. In any case, he will have to be on his knees and not with his legs stretched out, that is why we say that this position to have sex in the car has a small variation.

5. With legs raised

One posture that both of you will feel very comfortable with is that of the raised legs. To do this, they must be in the back seat and you must lie on your back in the chair with your legs raised, either resting them on your boy's shoulders, or resting your feet on the roof of the car.

6. Doggy pose

If they have time and are in a place where nobody can see them, they can also have sex in the car in the doggy style or the famous position on all fours. When they are in the back seat, get on all fours and your guy, leaning on his knee, can penetrate you from that angle. If they are in a place with a lot of privacy, they can even open the car door and your guy can stand outside of it to make it more comfortable for both of you.

In any case, what you really need to have sex in the car and be very satisfied are the desire, daring and creativity. You will see how they can manage at the moment.

The 10 sexual positions to get a deeper penetration.

Sex is a universe full of possibilities in which, once you have touched the right key, you are already the king of the game. But from time to time it is good to innovate, propose new things, try new sensibilities and sensations, that is why you should not say no to what your partner suggests (or vice versa). At the beginning of the year, it is a good excuse for you to explore something new in sex and thus the pleasure is greater. For example, deep penetration, a practice that if you are not very assiduous, we recommend that you try.

The deeper you go, the more pleasant and intense the sensation, which is fueled by the psychological arousal that comes from deep penetration. You will not argue that being deep inside a person warms the environment and even more the body. Therefore, for you to better experience this sensation, there are certain sexual positions that lend themselves much better to deep vaginal penetration. Take note and leave your partner with their mouths open the next time they play mambo.

1. Child's Pose (Balasana)

In this position, she sits on her heels and then leans forward with her arms extended forward and with her back straight. This variation of the doggy style allows full access to her vagina.

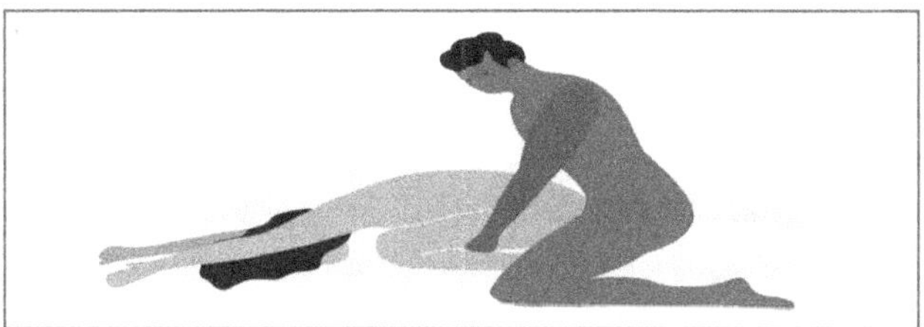

2. Iron

The woman lies on her stomach with her knees slightly bent and her hips slightly raised.

Keep your weight off her by supporting yourself with her arms (or if you like the feel of body and body, grab her by her hips and push from there).

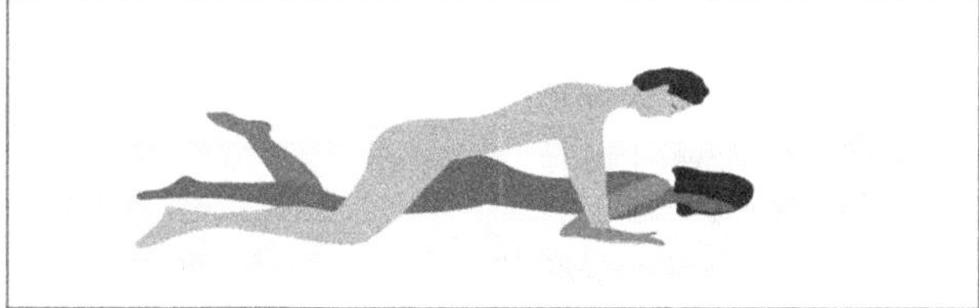

3. happy baby

Lying on your back, let the woman lift her legs bent and slightly apart at the height of her shoulders. For this pose to really work, she needs to grasp the soles of her feet with her hands.

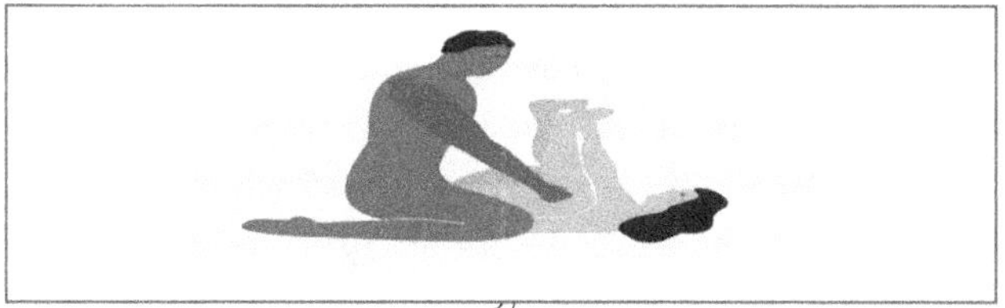

4. Legs on the shoulder

While she is on her back, have her place her legs on your shoulders so that the angle of her body should be approximately 90 degrees. The leg posture is what allows deep vaginal penetration. For more pleasure, push her pelvis up, slightly towards you.

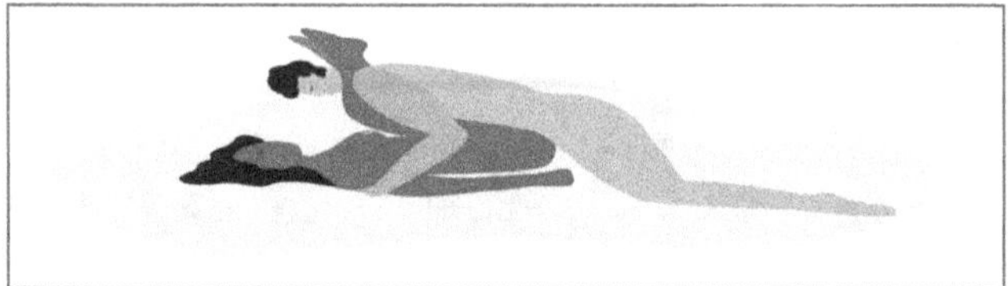

5. The Pearly Gates

While you are lying on your back, your partner lies on top of you with his back on your chest. From this position, it is also easy to stimulate her clitoris.

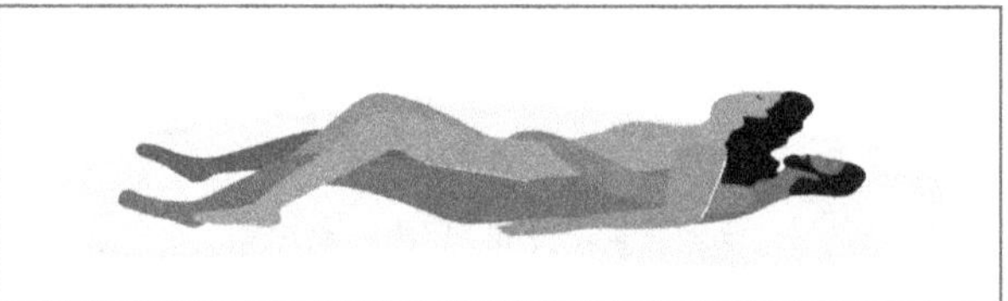

6. Kneel down and stand on your left leg while lying on your left side. From there, bend his right leg around the right side of your waist.

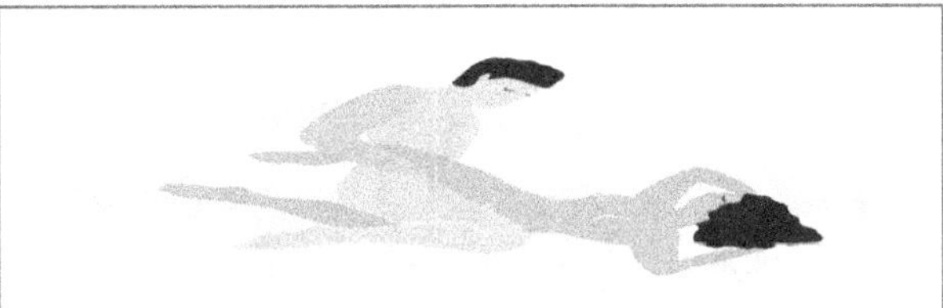

7. Wheelbarrow

Sit at the end of the bed and have your partner lie on his stomach with his hands on the floor in front of her with her vagina on your penis. This position might be a bit strenuous for her partner, but you can help her by holding most of her weight on you and only using her hands to steady yourself.

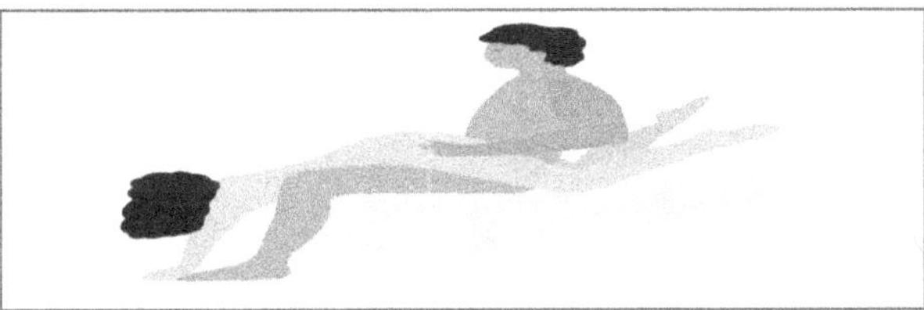

8. Teaspoon

This position is done with both of you lying on your side making the spoon. To increase the intensity, you can hug her tightly.

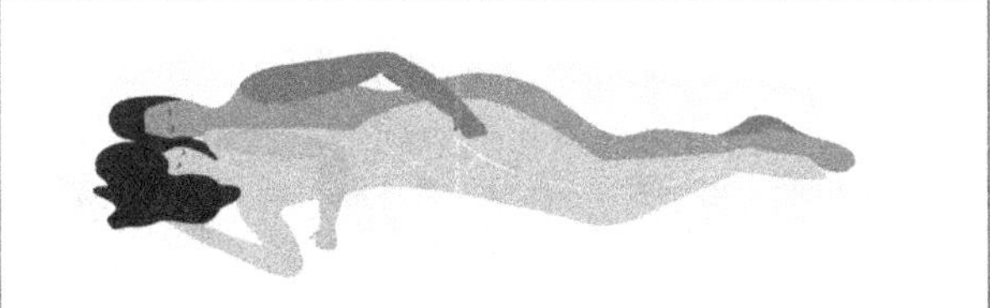

9. Lying down

Stand on the edge of the bed or a table while she lies back and lifts her legs toward her chest. You can also place her legs on your shoulders.

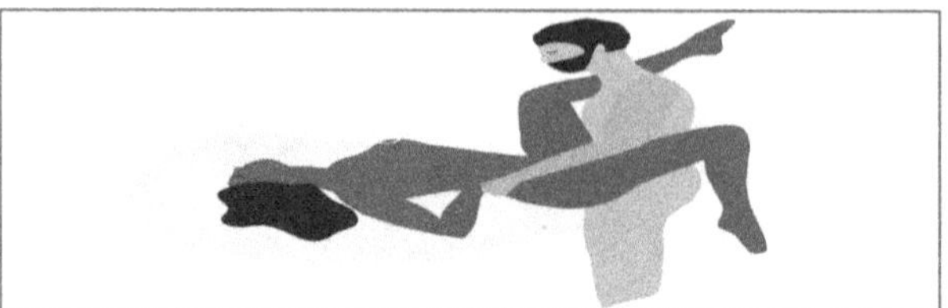

9. Missionary

Your partner lies on his back and you position yourself on top of him. Not only does this pose allow for deep penetration, but it is also a more intimate position, as you can kiss and maintain sustained eye contact while having sex.

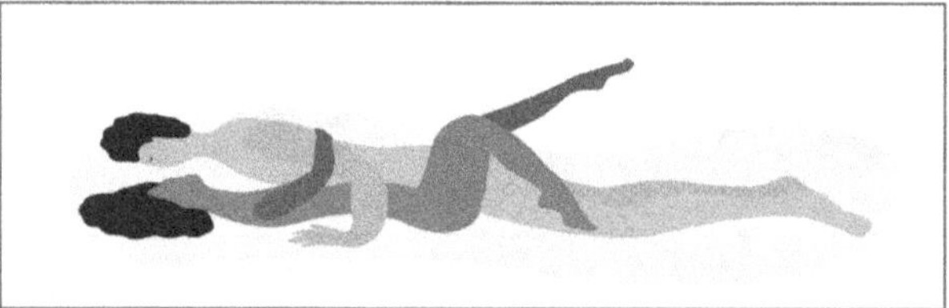

Tips for watching porn as a couple.

Have you ever wanted to propose to your partner, and you do not know how?

When we are determined to talk about something like this with our partner, we must be prepared. Even if you think that the trust and love between you will be enough to talk about the subject with total freedom, you should be careful: porn can bring out our insecurities, not just individual ones (with our body, image, or skill in the bed) but also within the relationship. Therefore, we recommend that, instead of jumping into the pool and finding that there is no water, keep these tips in mind.

1 - Speak it first.

In life it is always healthy to start by having a conversation. Have you ever watched porn? What type? What do you think about it? Is there anything that bothers you when you see it? The most important thing is to know the starting point, the experiences you have had with porn and how I felt when watching it. In that simple conversation, you will understand if your intentions have a future or not. Your partner may be afraid that you need to see other women men to get in tune with her in bed. Insecurities are the worst enemy of romantic relationships, and also of sexual ones. It is important that you reaffirm the relationship and make it understood that this is a shared experience to add pleasure and not a need.

If she doesn't want to, DON'T INSIST. You should not pressure your partner to do something they do not want to do, so before dropping the bomb in a conversation make sure they could be open to the idea and avoid putting them in an unnecessary commitment. If you decide to bring up the subject, you have to make him understand by all possible means that you do not want to put strange people in your bedroom (even if it is on video, the intrusion feels the same), but that this is just a tool to have fun and put a little of salsa in your sexual life. The words you choose are important.

2 - Do not go to the worst of the internet.

The key to being successful as a porn viewer is knowing where to turn. The first thing to understand is that pornography is not a list of monolithic movies that look the same and the same kind of people. Quite the contrary, there are a wide variety of film styles out there, you just have to find the one you like the most, from amateur porn to the more standard productions of Pornhub or feminist porn from authors like Erika Lust. Although from here we will always recommend betting on ethical porn. From there, we must look for what best suits us and not start with the prejudice that it does not matter because we are going to find the same thing wherever we go. That is not true.

If you are the one in charge of introducing porn to the couple and you throw a horrible video where there are violent attitudes or the actors seem to be having a hard time, most likely they do not want to try this experience anymore. Worse: surely, he will be left with a foreign body thinking that you like that. And whether it is so or not is something that does not interest us now. You must find something that you can both enjoy. We refer back to the first tip: talk about it. What if she tells you to choose? Surprise them? So, have it prepared in advance or be clear about where you want to go. Analyze how your partner is and put what you think could fit him. If you are a person who has seen porn before and is more open, take more risks. If you are a beginner and have already accepted a bit insecure, you probably want to visit the tag "for couples" or "for women" on more general websites or check alternative options such as Xconfessions or Lustery, where there is different material. The important thing is that you do not try to impose your tastes: make it a thing of two.

4 - Do not try to imitate everything you see.

There are times when porn could be classified as a sub-genre of fantasy. Wow, you don't have to believe everything. One of the most positive aspects of watching porn as a couple is the possibility of learning new things, of finding positions or movements that you would like to try on your own flesh. It is an inexhaustible source of ideas (if we know, as we said before, find the wealth of styles and stories) that can have sex less mechanical and monotonous. We all end up falling into vices that are good to break from time to time.

But at the same time, you must keep something in mind: porn is not perfect. Many times, it is even toxic. We can tend to forget that what we see on film is probably rehearsed, practiced by professionals (though not always), shot with a camera, and edited to create the final finish. That is, what we see is not 100% real. There is a staging, and, in certain films, there is also a completely falsified enjoyment. How many fake orgasms we have seen in porn. As many as in real life. Therefore, porn is routinely accused of building unrealistic expectations about sex, but it all needs to be put in context.

5 - Do not use it to fix something that is broken.

Sometimes we may think that it is okay to use porn as a way to spice up a sexual relationship that is somewhat faded, but the play can go very wrong. As we pointed out before, these types of experiences can very quickly bring out the frustrations of the couple, what you no longer fit in and that is leading the relationship to a standstill. Before trying this strategy, you should have a more in-depth, less sex-centric conversation, which generally raises more problems than solutions.

6 - Make it interactive.

If you stare too long without anything happening it can be weird. You have to avoid this situation, and it can be done in several ways: commenting on what is happening on the screen occasionally, stroking your partner subtly.

And, if things get hot enough, start the preliminaries while still watching the movie. That is, you do not have to pause and get into trouble. It is much more fun if you start little by little and following the rhythm of the actors, giving great importance to those caresses and various masturbations.

But beyond getting yourself in tune, it is important to comment on what you see. And there the words are also important again. Do not give orders (unless you discover that yours is dominance and submission in sex; that is another issue), it is better that you freely say what you like in what you are seeing and without a doubt your partner will pick up that suggestion to apply if it's something you feel comfortable with. Thus, through a more organic and less demanding conversation, no one will feel pressured to do something they do not want to do.

7 - Don't get used to it.

Watching porn every now and then is fine, but you should not get addicted or make your sex life dependent on it. Also, when something special becomes routine, that something stops being special. Or maybe you have set out to become the top porn experts in the country and your research must be intense. In general, and exceptions aside, it is recommended that it does not become a dependent habit and that you retain the ability to enjoy your bodies without any external help.

8 - Discuss it later.

If watching porn has inspired you to have a good time of sex and that is all you were looking for, great. But yes: do not forget to comment later. Yes, it seems that all we do is talk, but at some point, we will have to realize that in the conversation are the keys to having a healthier, more consensual, and happy sex life. You must talk about it before you know which way to go. We must talk during to identify what we like and that we might like to explore. And you have to talk later to find out how you have lived the experience and if you are open to repeating it. It is important to be honest, express your opinion without fear (but with respect) and seek that harmony with your partner.

9 798707 279225